Genomics for Nurses

This textbook introduces fundamental knowledge and the latest developments in genomics and explains their relevance to nursing practice, using case studies and activities to help readers to apply their learning. Genomics in health care is no longer limited to specialist areas or single genetic conditions. To provide holistic care, every practitioner in clinical practice now needs to know something about genomics.

This unique and timely text outlines what genomics is, and what it means for nurses. Among other issues it discusses:

- The UK context, including topics such as how genomics moves from research into practice and funding.
- Core nursing skills, alongside a discussion of where nurses are likely to be involved in patients' genomic journeys.
- Specific conditions and areas of practice where genomics is most relevant to nursing, with coverage of genetic testing, patient pathways and identification of risk.
- Ethics and genomics, including topics such as confidentiality, gene-editing and gene therapy, and resource allocation.
- Pharmacogenomics, and how an individual's genetic make-up can influence the efficacy of medical treatments.
- Future directions and challenges for the integration of genomics into healthcare practice.

Aligned with the relevant Nursing and Midwifery Council and NHS England competencies, it is an essential resource for nursing students and practising nurses.

Jodie Coulson is a lecturer in Prescribing and Medicines Optimisation at the University of York. She teaches pharmacology and has a special interest in pharmacogenomics. Jodie is currently working towards a PhD on Genomics in Nurse Education.

Genomics for Nurses

An Introduction

Jodie Coulson

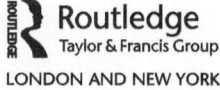

Routledge
Taylor & Francis Group

LONDON AND NEW YORK

Designed cover image: Getty Images

First published 2026
by Routledge
4 Park Square, Milton Park, Abingdon, Oxon OX14 4RN

and by Routledge
605 Third Avenue, New York, NY 10158

Routledge is an imprint of the Taylor & Francis Group, an informa business

British Library Cataloguing-in-Publication Data
A catalogue record for this book is available from the British Library

ISBN: 978-1-032-59121-6 (hbk)
ISBN: 978-1-032-59100-1 (pbk)
ISBN: 978-1-003-45304-8 (ebk)

DOI: 10.4324/9781003453048

Typeset in Sabon
by KnowledgeWorks Global Ltd.

This book is dedicated to my dad, Mick.

Contents

Acknowledgements

I would like to thank Sally Porter, who reads a lot and sends me interesting articles.

With thanks also to Helen Bethell and the NEY-GMSA for all the Lunch and Learns from which I learned a great deal.

This book would be worse without the good advice I received from Grace McInnes.

Thank you to Dr Ed Miller and Dr Emma Tonkin for including me in various interesting genomics opportunities.

I could not have written this book without support from Greg, who cooks when I want to work late, which is the sincerest form of love.

Glossary

Allele – An allele is one of two or more versions of a DNA sequence at a given genomic location. An individual inherits two alleles, one from each parent, for any given genomic location where such variation exists.

Aneuploidy – An abnormality in the number of chromosomes in a cell due to loss or duplication; any number of chromosomes other than the usual 46.

Autosomal dominant disorder – A pattern of inheritance characteristic of some genetic disorders. 'Autosomal' means that the gene in question is located on one of the non-sex chromosomes. 'Dominant' means that a single copy of the mutated gene (from one parent) is enough to cause the disorder. A child of a person affected by an autosomal dominant condition has a 50% chance of being affected by that condition via inheritance of a dominant allele.

Autosomal recessive disorder – A pattern of inheritance characteristic of some genetic disorders. 'Autosomal' means that the gene in question is located on one of the numbered, or non-sex chromosomes. 'Recessive' means that two copies of the mutated gene (one from each parent) are required to cause the disorder. In a family where both parents are carriers and do not have the disease, roughly a quarter of their children will inherit two disease-causing alleles and have the disease.

BRCA1 and BRCA2 genes – Genes associated with inherited forms of breast cancer and ovarian cancer. People with mutations in either BRCA1 or BRCA2 have a much higher risk for developing breast, ovarian or other types of cancer than those without mutations in the genes. Both BRCA1 and BRCA2 normally act as tumour suppressors, meaning that they help to regulate cell division. Most people have two active copies of these genes. When one of the two copies becomes inactive owing to an inherited mutation, a person's cells are left with only one copy. If this remaining copy also becomes inactivated, then uncontrolled cell growth results, which leads to breast, ovarian or other types of cancer.

The Central dogma of molecular biology – A theory stating that genetic information flows only in one direction, from DNA, to RNA, to protein, or from RNA directly to protein.

Chromosomes – Structures made of protein and a single molecule of DNA which carry the genomic information from cell to cell. Humans have 22 pairs of numbered chromosomes (autosomes) and one pair of sex chromosomes (XX or XY), for a total of 46 in the nucleus of each cell. Each pair contains two chromosomes, one coming from each parent, which means that children inherit half of their chromosomes from their mother and half from their father.

CRISPR – Clustered regularly interspaced short palindromic repeats – a technology used by research scientists to selectively modify the DNA.

DNA – Deoxyribonucleic acid – the molecule that carries genetic information for the development and functioning of an organism. It is made from two linked strands that wind around each other to form a double helix. Each strand has a backbone made of alternating sugar (deoxyribose) and phosphate groups. Attached to each sugar is one of four bases: adenine (A), cytosine (C), guanine (G) or thymine (T). The two strands are connected by chemical bonds between the bases: adenine bonds with thymine and cytosine bonds with guanine. The sequence of the bases along DNA's backbone encodes biological information, such as the instructions for making a protein or RNA molecule.

Epigenetics – Modifications to DNA structure which do not change the DNA sequence but can affect gene expression. Modifications can be inherited or occur within the lifespan. Modifications may include chemical modification or methylation.

Exome – The exome comprises about 2% of the genome in the form of exons which contain the genetic code for proteins.

Gene – A DNA sequence that contains the code or biological instructions for the production of a polypeptide chain, usually a specific protein or component of a protein.

Genetic code – The instructions contained in a gene that tell a cell how to make a specific protein. The code within each gene uses sequences of the four nucleotide bases (adenine, cytosine, guanine, and thymine) to specify which amino acid is needed at each position within a protein.

Genome – An organism's complete set of DNA or genetic material, including coding and non-coding regions.

Gene expression – The process by which the information encoded in a gene is used to direct the assembly of a protein molecule. This mostly occurs via the transcription of RNA molecules that code for proteins. Gene expression is thought of as an 'on/off switch' to control when and where RNA molecules and proteins are made. The process of gene expression is carefully regulated, changing substantially under different conditions.

Genotype – The DNA sequence of an organism or individual, which determines in combination with environmental influences the specific characteristics (phenotype) of an organism or person.

GMSAs – Genomic medicine service alliances – a network of regional support services supporting the integration of genomics within the UK NHS.

HER2 – Human epidermal growth factor receptor 2 – a protein involved in cell growth which can be overexpressed in cancers such as breast cancer. The presence of HER2 can help determine treatment options.

Lynch syndrome – An inherited condition or pre-cancer syndrome which increases the risk of developing some cancers, including colorectal cancer. It is sometimes called hereditary non-polyposis colorectal cancer.

Methylation – The addition of methyl groups to DNA which can affect gene expression and the production of proteins for which the gene encodes.

MMR gene – Mismatch repair genes correct errors occurring during in DNA replication. Can be inactivated leading to impaired DNA repair and cell mutations, which can increase the risk of cancer.

mRNA – Messenger ribonucleic acid – carries genetic information form the cell nucleus into the cytoplasm, to be interpreted by ribosomes to make proteins.

NGS – Next generation sequencing – a DNA sequencing technology which can process large volumes of DNA.

Oncogene – Proto oncogenes regulate cell division and mutations in these genes which change them into oncogenes can cause cells to divide unchecked and have the potential to cause cancer.

Pedigree – A term sometimes used to mean family health history or family tree.

Pharmacogenomics – Combines pharmacology and genomics to predict individual responses to certain medicines and improve treatment outcomes.

Phenotype – An individual's observable physical characteristics directly influenced by the genotype and/or environment. This can include the observed signs and symptoms of a genetic or genomic condition.

Polygenic risk score – A calculation to determine risk levels for complex or polygenic disease using information concerning inherited and environmental contributors.

RNA – Ribonucleic acid – the product of DNA transcription.

Single nucleotide polymorphisms (SNPs) – Variation of a single base pair at a specific location within the DNA. Can influence health, contribute to disease and affect an individual's response to some medications.

Some entries have been adapted from glossaries provided by the National Human Genome Research Institute and the Genomics Education Programme

What is genomics?

Chapter outline
This chapter explains what genomics is and outlines how genomics is relevant to nursing practice. It also contains a review of the structure and function of DNA and describes gene expression and the inheritance patterns of common genetic conditions. This chapter considers how advances in genomic science and technologies, the increased availability of genomic tests and the translation of genomic information into care will affect the nursing role and the skills required to perform this role.

In each chapter of this book, there are learning activities linked to the NHS England 2023 Genomic Competency Framework for UK Nurses and links to further resources to extend your knowledge of genomics.

Introduction

Genomics is the study of genes and their functions including inherited changes and changes caused by environmental factors (World Health Organization, 2025). As new technologies and our understanding of the genetic and genomic basis of disease develop, the nursing role is expanding to include care of patients as part of their genomics journeys. The Nursing and Midwifery Council (NMC, 2018, p.11) states that at the point of registration, nurses must be able to demonstrate knowledge of genomics as a determinant of health.

Most nurses, nurse associates and student nurses can think of examples of care related to the many genetic or hereditary conditions caused by variations in single genes, or 'monogenic' conditions, such as cystic fibrosis, haemochromatosis and sickle cell anaemia. For example, people with cystic fibrosis may have regular contact with health services to review their medication or to treat chest infections. However, in addition to monogenic conditions, genes are now also understood to

DOI: 10.4324/9781003453048-1

contribute to most common diseases and complex or multifactorial health conditions such as heart disease, stroke, diabetes, some cancers, Alzheimer's disease, chronic respiratory conditions and autoimmune conditions (Tonkin and Skirton, 2013). Such conditions occur owing to inherited variations in our genes combined with changes to our genes across the lifespan caused by lifestyle and environmental factors such as diet and smoking.

Genes are responsible for how we respond to infectious diseases caused by viruses and bacteria and can also determine how we will respond to some medicines (Tluczek et al., 2019). Technology has developed to enable health practitioners to test for abnormalities in a person's genes, which they have inherited from their parents. Genetic variants are locations where the genetic code looks slightly different from normal, for example the sequence might be in a different order, or a part may be missing. Looking for differences in specific genes can identify variants a person was born with which mean that they are more susceptible to developing certain conditions. For example, inherited changes in the cells which make up the respiratory system may mean that a person is more vulnerable to developing problems such as chronic obstructive pulmonary disorder (COPD). This information enables nurses to give information about how a person can protect themselves from the risk of developing COPD, including avoiding or stopping smoking, which causes inflammatory changes more quickly and more severely in persons with specific inherited genetic variations (Tamimi et al., 2012).

As the largest professional group in health care systems and a primary contact for many patients, nurses have an important role in the interpretation of genetic information relevant to patient care (World Health Organization, 2025). Information about any genetic vulnerabilities a person may have inherited can help nurses to recommend screening for specific variants and this can take place sooner than screening tests offered to the general population. Obtaining information about how their genetic configuration might determine their future health enables people to make guided decisions which are likely to improve their health outcomes. For example, if a person is aware that one or more members of their family have a BRCA gene variation, which can lead to breast cancer and some other cancers including ovarian, pancreatic and prostate cancer, they can test to see if they have the same variant. This may pre-empt regular screening and if tests are positive, they may be offered preventive or prophylactic treatment.

New therapies and treatment modalities have been developed through advances in genomics technologies (Buaki-Sogo and Percival, 2022). For example, tests can be performed to identify changes to the genetic code which have occurred over time and are affecting cellular function in some organs. Some changes to genes which occur through exposure to environmental harms such as pollution can affect cell growth. Tumours are caused by unregulated cell growth, and it is possible to test the DNA in the nuclei of tumour cells to determine the best way to treat them. Precision oncology is an area within which genomics has developed quickly towards reducing the time to diagnosis and improving prognosis, and nurses have played a significant role in developing services around testing and ongoing care to realise the potential of new genomics technologies for patients (Calzone et al., 2018).

Some people respond differently to some forms of chemotherapy, for example fluoro-pyrimidines, owing to common genetic variations or *polymorphisms* in certain genes, and nurses also have a vital role in using genomic information to improve medicines' safety. Pharmacogenomic tests can be performed to predict whether a person might be at increased risk of harm from a medicine and this information can inform dose adjustment and careful monitoring to prevent avoidable harm.

This book explores genomics in nursing practice and the skills involved in genomic proficiency for nurses. It aims to provide insight into what all nurses need to know about genomics, including the identification of genetic and genomic risk. Information is provided about the current UK genomics testing infrastructure and ethical issues associated with genomic tests. The skills required of those working in specialist genomics areas and the nursing role in understanding how individual responsiveness or reactions to some medicines can contribute to the efficacy and safety of some treatments are also explored.

So, what exactly is genomics?

The World Health Organization (2020) defines genetics as the study of heredity and genomics as a field of science that studies the function of genes, the relationships between them and the combined influence of these factors on human development. The National Human Genome Research Institute (2019) differentiates between genetics as the study of individual genes and genomics as the study of the entire genome. The genome is all of an organism's genetic material and genomics concerns interactions between genes, and the effects of environmental factors on genes. Environmental factors include not only those within the physical environment but also lifestyle, cultural and psychosocial influences. These elements can affect *gene expression,* which means when genes are switched on or switched off, specifically the expression of genes relating to cell growth and repair.

Genomic medicine involves working with available information from a person's genome to try to improve their health outcomes. For many, a genetic diagnosis can provide the answer to long-term symptoms or health problems. Achieving an accurate diagnosis, at a molecular level, underpins better targeted treatment options which can lead to more effective therapeutic outcomes. Testing for cell changes early and prescribing treatment or taking other action as soon as possible, for example if there is prostate cancer in a man's family, can have a significant positive impact. Inherited variation in single genes which increase risks to health is also considered in the context of a person's everyday life to give a fuller picture of their overall current and likely future health. Exploring lifestyle behaviours and any exposure to carcinogenic substances or pollutants, which can precipitate pathogenic changes or mutations, can help to more accurately predict the level or extent of genomic risk.

Genomic testing can improve the speed and accuracy of diagnosis for many conditions, including rare inherited conditions. Child developmental delay is also often found to have a genetic cause. Genomics enables health care professionals to better understand the underlying causes of disease, which helps them to provide better information to patients and better care (Buaki-Sogo and Percival, 2022).

Within health care, the term genomics is now used to include care related to genomic testing, diagnosis and treatment. It also refers to factors affecting health caused by variations in *any part* of the genome, across the lifespan; this includes coding genes or the instructions that make us who we are, which make up only about 1% of our genetic material (*the exome*), in addition to non-coding genes and other structural matter. Genomics also concerns the parts of our DNA which cause genes to be switched on or off at certain points – the regulatory sequences that control gene expression. Information from the whole genome can reveal whether some people may be more likely to develop some diseases in later life such as Parkinson's disease or Alzheimer's disease.

Advances in genomics mean that the nursing role must evolve and adapt to new scientific understanding and new elements of care. Nurses who understand the genetic–genomic contribution to health and disease are vital in realising the impact of genomic technological advances on treatment and care (Greco and Salveson, 2009). Many current services reflect accurate predictions that the nursing community will eventually be able to use genomics for health promotion and disease prevention, diagnosis, prescription and the monitoring of treatment (Calzone et al., 2010; Daack-Hirsch et al., 2011).

Genes, DNA and chromosomes

The nucleus of every cell in the human body includes 2 metres of DNA (deoxyribonucleic acid), which contains sequences of genes or the *genetic code* for the composition and function of the entire organism. The code comprises instructions which tell each individual cell what type of cell to be and how to behave, including the regulation of its own growth, reproduction and death (Cancer Research UK, 2023). There are many different cells in the body with singular functions according to the tissue, organ and body system they belong to. For example, in the respiratory system, the trachea or airway has several types of cells that are structured differently and perform different roles. Goblet cells secrete mucous to trap and expel inhaled particles and pathogens and smooth muscle cells line the airways and can relax to cause dilatation or the opening of the airway at times when a person needs to take in more oxygen, for example when they exercise.

Genes are made from pairs of single nucleotide bases (guanine, adenine, thymine and cytosine) and the human genome comprises three billion base pairs. Guanine always pairs with cytosine and adenine pairs with thymine. These base pairs form a pre-determined sequence for the grouping of amino acids to create proteins such as the components of cells, enzymes and hormones that make up the human body (National Human Genome Research Institute, 2019.)

Within cell nuclei, strands of DNA are wound around structural histones, like spools, and 'packaged' into *chromosomes* (Figure 1.1). In a person's body, each cell nucleus contains 23 pairs of chromosomes with one from their biological mother and one from their biological father making up each pair (Figure 1.2). Twenty-two of the pairs (autosomes) carry information for physical functions and characteristics aside from biological sex. Pair 23 is the sex chromosomes which determine whether a person is born as biologically male or female. A person's biological father has an X-chromosome and a Y-chromosome, and their mother has two X-chromosomes. A child who inherits an X-chromosome from their mother and the Y-chromosome from their father will be male, whereas a female child will inherit an X-chromosome from their mother and their father's X-chromosome.

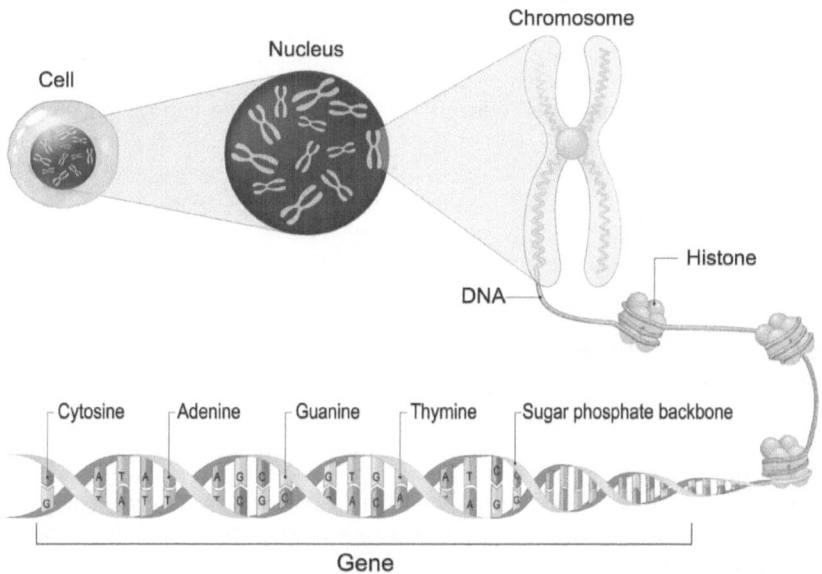

Figure 1.1 The structure of DNA.

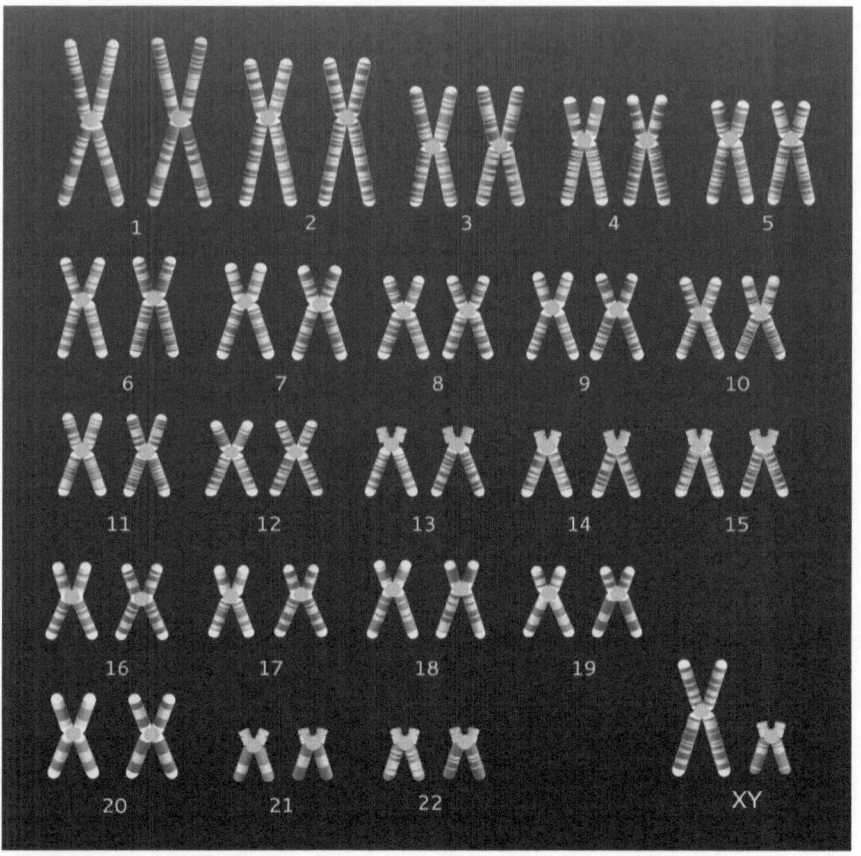

Figure 1.2 The human karyotype.

Gene expression

The genes that code for specific proteins can be active or inactive (expressed or not expressed) at certain points in a person's development and across their lifespan. For example, genes that regulate growth and development are active at different times to the genes that cause ageing. Gene expression refers to how, where and when the information or code within a gene is turned into a function (National Human Genome Research Institute, 2019).

When genes are expressed, they guide the formation of essential physiological proteins. Proteins are made using the core principle or *central dogma* of molecular biology (Figure 1.3). This principle describes the process in which DNA copies or transcribes the genetic code (the instructions to make proteins) into RNA. Messenger RNA (mRNA) carries the code outside of the cell nucleus to be read or translated by ribosomes. Amino acids form chains, according to the translated instructions, to make a functional protein (Lesk, 2017). Insulin, for example, is a hormone, made up of two chains of amino acids, required to regulate blood glucose levels.

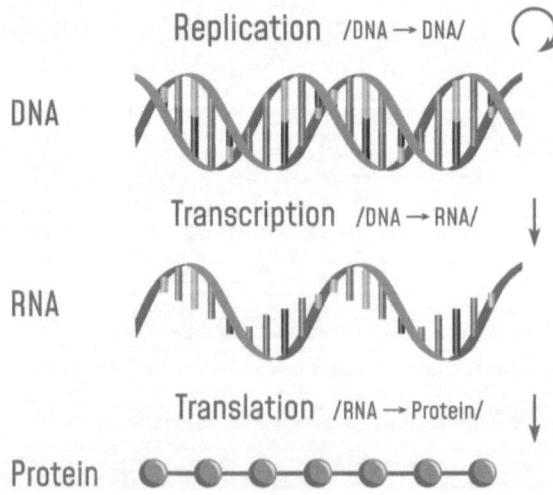

Figure 1.3 The central dogma of molecular biology.

> ### 🧁 The central dogma of molecular biology made easy
>
> 1. Transcription – Polly brings muffins to work which she baked using her Granny Dina's recipe. Polly's colleague Robert loves the muffins and asks for the recipe, so Polly *copies* it down for him and brings it to work the next day. Robert has a day off, so Polly gives the recipe to Ryan, who lives near to Robert, to pop it through his letterbox on the way home.
>   *In the cell nucleus, the enzyme polymerase transfers information (codes for specific proteins) from DNA strands to RNA. Messenger RNA (mRNA) carries the code from the nucleus into the cell.*
> 2. Translation – on Saturday, Robert buys some ingredients and prepares to bake. Robert reads through the copy of Granny Dina's recipe to *understand* how to make the muffins and measures out the ingredients.
>   *Ribosomes translate the genetic code in the RNA.*
> 3. Replication – Robert follows the step-by-step instructions to make the new muffins which turn out just the same as Granny Dina's
>   *Long polypeptide chains of amino acids (forming new proteins) are synthesised.*

Gene expression determines the characteristics or traits of an individual such as their hair or eye colour. There are different patterns of inheritance which different genes typically follow. A person's *genotype* refers to their individual genetic information or code, including any variation within particular *alleles* or variations in genes at a specific location which determine individual characteristics or traits. Alleles are different versions of the same gene within which inherited variation is expected to occur (Tonkin and Skirton, 2013). Corresponding alleles from each parent appear in the same place on each chromosome in a pair and contain the information contributing to an individual's unique and varied characteristics. Normal genetic differences, between individuals represent places in the genetic code where allelic variation can appear and the resulting traits, like eye colour, can be displayed in a number of different ways.

Some genes are *dominant* which means that when a particular allele is present it will be expressed, and this expression will result in a specific trait (like brown eyes). Some genes are *recessive* (like the allele for blue eyes), which means that they may not be expressed when paired with a dominant allele. When a recessive gene is not expressed, a person will not show the particular trait which that gene codes for. The arrangement of all the genetic material passed down by both parents, which they inherited from their own parents, grandparents and so on, will determine a person's eye colour, hair colour and blood type. More complex characteristics such as skin colour involve the interaction of multiple alleles, and this interaction is what causes each of us to look unique.

Genes from both parents will determine whether a trait is dominant or recessive and the theoretical probability of inheriting a particular trait can be charted based on these familial genotypes. Dominant genes include the genes for dark hair and for blood type A. Punnett squares can be used as a visual representation of the likelihood of any child receiving the alleles that cause specific traits to be inherited from their parents. Punnett squares use Mendelian (after Gregor Mendel who discovered them) principles

EYE COLOUR GENETICS

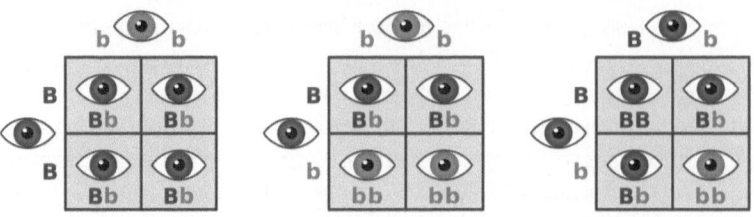

B - DOMINANT BROWN EYE ALLELE
b - RECESSIVE BLUE EYE ALLELE

Figure 1.4 Punnett squares depicting inheritance patterns for eye colour.

of inheritance to predict the possible eye colour (Figure 1.4) or blood type of a child when the genotypes of both parents are known.

Punnett squares can also show parents the probability of a child inheriting a genetic variant which may cause them to be affected by or to be a carrier for a specific genetic condition. In autosomal dominant conditions, only one faulty copy of a gene is required for a child to be affected by the condition. In autosomal recessive conditions like Sickle cell disease a faulty copy must be inherited from each parent and inheriting only one faulty copy means that the child will be a carrier for the condition but not affected by it. The sickle cell Punnett square (Figure 1.5) shows the likelihood, if both parents are carriers for sickle cell trait but not affected by the disease, of any of their children being born with sickle cell trait (2/4), with sickle cell disease (1/4) or unaffected (1/4).

The genotype refers to the inherited code for a trait, but a person's *phenotype* is the term used to describe the outward presentation, or observable traits, which can be influenced and changed. Changes in phenotype may be caused by the interaction of a person's genotype with their environment. For example, the code for a particular skin colour can be inherited but skin can become darker in colour following exposure to the sun and the increased production of melanin.

Some factors can affect or override genetic inheritance patterns to determine whether a gene is expressed at a certain time. For example, particular genes might only be expressed under certain environmental conditions such as specific humidity and oxygen levels when homeostatic adaptations in the body affect hormonal and metabolic

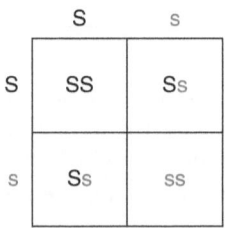

Figure 1.5 Punnet square depicting inheritance patterns for sickle cell disease and sickle cell trait.

processes. Pollution, radiation or exposure to certain chemicals such as pesticides or those in materials like asbestos can also influence gene expression (Lesk, 2017). Cigarette smoke, processed foods, lack of physical activity and stress can also have an impact. Gene expression changes as people age and the extent to which certain genes are expressed or not expressed can affect both physical, for example by influencing muscle strength, and cognitive function (Harris et al., 2017.)

How genetics determine health

Genetic disease is caused by mutations or variations in the genetic code which affect a person's health. The main types of genetic disease are:

- chromosomal disorders
- single gene disorders
- complex disorders

Chromosomal disorders

Chromosomal disorders are caused by differences in the number or structure of an individual's chromosomes and are not usually inherited but caused by random changes during foetal development (Shaw and Lurie, 2023). Aneuploidy is a type of chromosomal abnormality, and this term is used to describe conditions in which cells have an abnormal number of chromosomes. Down syndrome (trisomy 21) is an example of aneuploidy and people with Down syndrome have an extra copy of Chromosome 21. Other examples include Patau syndrome (trisomy 13), Edwards' syndrome (trisomy 18) and Turner Syndrome.

📖 **Knowledge focus – Turner syndrome**

- Turner syndrome occurs randomly and affects 1 in every 2000 baby girls.
- Girls with Turner syndrome inherit only one normal copy of the X-chromosome.
- Turner syndrome usually causes under-development of the ovaries, resulting in a lack of menses.
- Turner syndrome may not be recognised until puberty.
- Girls with Turner syndrome are usually also a shorter than average height.
- There is no cure, but associated symptoms can be treated, for example with growth hormone therapy and oestrogen and progesterone replacement theory.
- Although most women will remain infertile, if their womb has developed successfully, IVF pregnancies can be a successful option when somebody who is affected by Turner syndrome wishes to start a family (NHS, 2021).

Single gene disorders

Some conditions can be caused by unpredictable variations in specific alleles or 'errors' in the genetic code. These variations can appear in the ordering of the sequences, or as the deletion or duplication of a section of DNA which can affect the structure and function of the genes in these areas. Variations in a person's genes will be passed on to their children if they appear in the DNA which a child inherits from them. When a genetic variation or variant appears in a known location and causes previously identified associated symptoms then it may be possible, in combination with other clinical information, to diagnose a genetic condition. For example, Tay–Sachs disease is a monogenic condition caused by variation in a single gene. This degenerative condition is inherited in an autosomal recessive pattern which means that when both parents are carriers of the same variant in the HEXA gene, each of their children has a one in four chance of developing the condition. Infants with Tay–Sachs disease lack a specific protein which can cause damage to the brain and spinal cord that worsens over time. They have mobility, hearing and visual problems. Other inherited genetic conditions caused by variations in single genes disorders include cystic fibrosis, Huntington's disease, Duchenne muscular dystrophy and polycystic kidney disease.

The recessive and dominant inheritance patterns for particular traits were discovered in the nineteenth century by Gregor Mendel experimenting on pea plants. Pathological or disease-causing genetic variations are often inherited in the same way. Simple monogenetic inheritance patterns include:

- autosomal dominant inheritance
- autosomal recessive inheritance
- X-linked inheritance
- mitochondrial (maternal) inheritance

Children are born with autosomal dominant conditions when they inherit only one copy of the disease-causing gene from either parent (Figure 1.6). The parent with the faulty gene will also have the condition. Each of their children has a 50% chance of inheriting the variant gene and of developing the disease or of inheriting the healthy copy, in addition to a healthy copy from the unaffected parent and not developing the disease. Autosomal dominant conditions are so called because the variant which causes them appears on one of the autosomes or non-sex chromosomes. They tend to appear in most generations of a family and examples include Huntington's disease, osteogenesis imperfecta (brittle bones) and Marfan syndrome.

When a child is born with an autosomal recessive condition a variant copy of the same gene (with the same variant) is inherited from both parents (Figure 1.6). Two copies of a disease-causing variant are needed for a child to have this type of disorder. Examples include cystic fibrosis, sickle cell disease and Tay–Sachs disease. Because the genetic variants for these conditions are recessive or hidden when inherited alongside a healthy copy of the gene from the other parent, individuals may not know they are carriers for these conditions, and the conditions may not manifest in every generation.

X-Linked conditions are caused by inherited faults from either parent on an X-chromosome (Figure 1.6). Fathers cannot pass X-linked traits to their sons (there is no male-to-male transmission), because all sons inherit only the Y-chromosome from their father and an X-chromosome from their mother. X-Linked gene variants can be inherited in a dominant or a recessive pattern. Females are more frequently affected than males because they have two X-chromosomes, but males tend to be more severely affected by these conditions because they only have one X-chromosome. Females who inherit X-linked genetic variants have a normal copy of the variant gene on their second

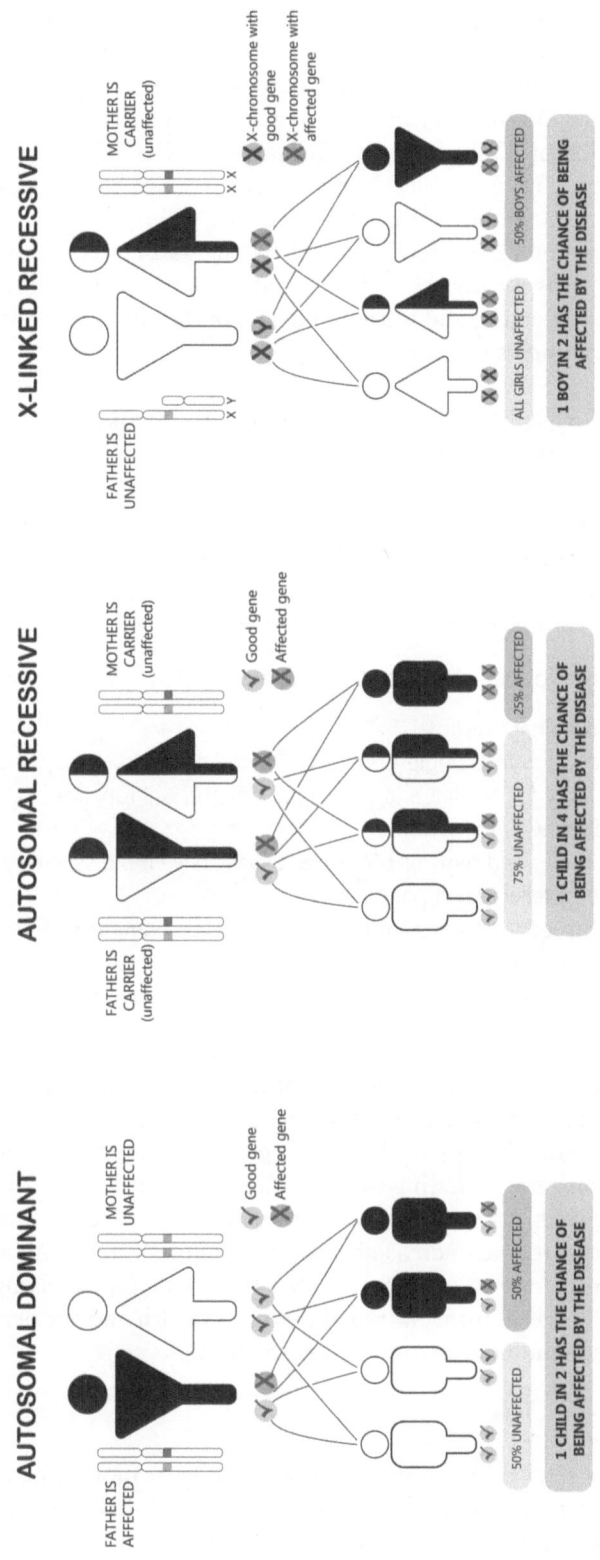

Figure 1.6 Autosomal dominant, autosomal recessive and x-linked recessive inheritance patterns.

X-chromosome to counterbalance any loss of function. Examples of X-linked conditions include Duchenne muscular dystrophy and fragile X syndrome (Genetic Alliance, 2025).

Mitochondria are cellular organelles which use oxygen and glucose from the blood to produce energy (ATP) for cell function. Mitochondrial diseases are conditions which affect the production of ATP and the performance of cells, tissues organs and body systems. Gene variants leading to mitochondrial diseases can be X-linked or non-X-linked (the variant can appear on an autosome or on the X-chromosome) and when they are X-linked, males are more severely affected by the associated disorder than females. Only females can pass on mitochondrial conditions to their children but both males and females can be affected, and mitochondrial conditions can appear in every generation of a family. Examples include:

- mitochondrial encephalopathy, lactic acidosis and stroke-like episodes syndrome
- Leber hereditary optic neuropathy
- Leigh syndrome
- Kearns–Sayre syndrome
- myoclonic epilepsy and ragged-red fibre disease

📖 Knowledge focus – fragile X Syndrome (FXS)

- an X-linked dominant disorder;
- caused by variation in a single gene (FMR1) leading to deficiency of a specific protein (FMRP) necessary for normal brain development and cell function;
- a neurodevelopmental syndrome;
- affects both males and females but males usually have more severe symptoms;
- usually causes intellectual impairment;
- associated with behavioural symptoms such as ADHD and anxiety and sometimes irritability and aggression;
- strong links to autism spectrum disorder (Richter and Zhao, 2021).

A person's ancestry can affect their risk of inheriting a specific genetic vulnerability owing to the increased prevalence of some genetic variants within some ethnic groups. For example, one mutated copy of the BRCA gene can significantly increase the risk of developing some cancers, including breast cancer, and BRCA gene mutations are more prevalent in those with African and Ashkenazi Jewish ethnic ancestry (Calzone et al., 2010). When a person is at increased risk of developing a specific condition, genetic tests can obtain information from their DNA from a biological sample, such as blood or saliva, which can reveal information about their health and the health of their family (National Human Genome Research Institute, 2019).

Complex disorders

Complex disorders refer to pathologies caused by one or more genetic variants in combination with environmental factors, for example Type 2 diabetes. Inherited gene mutations can affect the expression of the gene which regulates pancreatic β-cell function and the production of insulin. Diabetes is a metabolic disease caused by a lack of insulin. Insulin is required to facilitate the entry of glucose into cells and low levels of insulin can cause high blood glucose levels (hyperglycaemia) and associated harms, for example cardiovascular disease, peripheral neuropathy and kidney damage. In combination with inherited variations which can affect glucose regulation and increase a person's susceptibility to developing type 2 diabetes, environmental or lifestyle factors such as infrequent physical activity can cause changes to insulin production or resistance to the effects of insulin and greatly increase the risk of harm. Type 2 diabetes manifests differently in different individuals but can have a significant impact on health (Hu et al., 2020).

Epigenetics

Epigenetics is concerned with the impact of environmental and lifestyle factors on gene expression. Epigenetic modification can occur as a result of damage to cells and does not change DNA sequences themselves but influences how the body interprets these instructions and how genes are expressed. These changes can alter cell growth and development and negatively affect a person's health. Because some epigenetic changes are caused by modifiable behaviours, nurses can promote protective measures such as a healthy diet and reduced alcohol consumption to improve health and reduce risk. There is a significant relationship between diet, gene expression and health outcomes with appropriate nutritional intake contributing to better gut health, improved circadian rhythms and decreased susceptibility to disease (Prasad et al., 2011).

Detrimental changes to health, including malnutrition and obesity, can be precipitated by intrinsic socio-economic factors and health disparities, and for some individuals it may be more difficult for nurses to initiate interventions which result in lasting change. Nursing responsibilities involve recognising health risks, promoting health and providing adequate patient education to the best of their ability and in cases where this proves challenging, developing skills and knowledge in this area can enhance practice (Calzone et al., 2010). Researching specific conditions can help to increase knowledge of common late-onset diseases for example age-related macular degeneration. This is a condition in which the accumulation of lipid and protein deposits in the retina leads to retinal degeneration and visual impairment. This condition is generally caused by genetic variants which affect lipid metabolism and exacerbated by environmental factors such as smoking and a diet low in antioxidants (found in leafy vegetables). Information from the genome, combined with information supplied by patients regarding diet, can support nurses with appropriate knowledge to explore effective preventative care (Swaroop et al., 2009).

Psychosocial factors causing changes to health include minimal motivation to exercise, reduced social contact and substance misuse. Environmental harms, including poor air quality where patients live and exposure to diseases and viruses can also cause epigenetic changes in some individuals. When genes are not expressed (inhibited), they do not fulfil their intended function. Many gene mutations are known to be caused by exposure to environmental stressors, including those which lead to the development of some cancers, including lung cancer, bladder cancer and colorectal cancer. When the mismatch repair (MMR) gene, which detects and checks abnormal cell growth is not expressed, abnormal cells such as tumour cells can grow freely. The MMR gene can be switched off by an inherited gene variation or as a result of epigenetic changes (Mbemi et al., 2020).

Pre-natal stress factors and experiences in early childhood can also cause changes to the epigenome, which can influence gene expression and affect child learning and development. Traumatic early life experiences can leave chemical markers on genes referred to as DNA *methylation*. Nurses can work with parents to promote a healthy lifestyle, adequate socialisation and appropriate learning opportunities to support genomic health (Harvard University Center on the Developing Child, 2019).

The benefits of genomics technologies for patients

The benefits of genomic medicine for improving health are outlined by NHS England (2022) and include:

- early diagnosis
- more precise diagnosis
- more effective treatments
- fewer adverse reactions
- eligibility for clinical trials
- prognostics and preventative approaches

📖 **Learning activity**

- Think of some different patients or patient groups with whom you have come into contact who might have accessed or would benefit from accessing genomic services as part of their care.

(This learning activity is linked to NHS England (2023) genomic nursing competency 1.)

Whole genome sequencing

The Human Genome Project which ran between 1990 and 2003 was a study within which an international group of researchers studied DNA given by anonymous volunteers around the world. In April of 2003, scientists were able to publish the full sequence of the human genome or the complete set of human DNA (National Human Genome Research Institute, 2024). It is now possible to screen the whole genome of an individual and compare it with the published sequence to identify potentially harmful inherited or spontaneous variations and epigenetic changes. Whole genome sequencing is currently offered to some specific patient groups in England and Wales, for example to reach a diagnosis for those with undiagnosed or rare diseases and for adults and children with some types of cancer, including some cancers of the blood.

The Generation Study (previously the Newborn Screening Programme) was launched by Genomics England in 2023. This study is an NHS research project which aims to understand whether sequencing the whole genomes of neonates could help to discover more rare genetic conditions earlier in life. The study is screening participants for 223 individual conditions caused by over 500 different genes. The selected conditions were chosen because tests will provide a clear result (they are conditions which have been previously identified and linked to a specific variant), they are treatable and early treatment will improve quality of life. It is expected that approximately 1% of those screened will be diagnosed with a genetic condition and that a diagnosis will improve their health outcomes. Education is provided for the nurses and other health care professionals who will be involved in a person's ongoing care when a condition is identified through this research (Genomics England, 2024).

Genomic data from participants will be added to the established evidence base and contribute to the progression of genomic science. Data from the trial will be used to ascertain:

- how mapping the genetic code at birth will affect the lifetime health of individuals;
- whether newborn screening can be implemented at scale;
- how genomic data can be used to improve and develop new diagnostic tests and treatments; and
- the risks and benefits of storing genomic data over a person's lifetime (Horton et al., 2024).

The BabySeq project is an equivalent study in the US which also began in 2023. This study is purposefully recruiting participants from families who self-identify as Black/African American or Hispanic/Latino to make up more than 50% of participants. This is a key aspect of the design of the study, which aims to improve the diversity of the data obtained and the usefulness of the research for all (Smith et al., 2024).

Whole exome screening can also be used for the early detection of genetic disorders. Screening just the *exome* or protein coding part of the genome, where most variations associated with disease occur, is quicker and more cost effective. Foetal exome screening can be requested for high-risk pregnancies including pregnancies for which an ultrasound scan has shown suspected genetic abnormalities. Rapid exome screening is useful when neonates present with symptoms suggestive of a genetic condition and have been admitted to a neo-natal intensive care unit. This type of test can quickly inform decision-making and clinical management (D'Gama et al., 2022). Genomics in obstetrics and gynaecology is explored further in Chapter 2.

Genome-wide association studies

Genome-wide association studies (GWASs) involve scanning the genomes of a large cohort of participants who have a genetic condition and a control group who do not have the condition. This data collection and comparison technique helps researchers to understand the genetic and genomic variants associated with specific common and rare disorders. It can help them to understand which genetic variations do not cause disease. It can also help to better understand individual variation in the quality and severity of symptoms linked to different diseases, including the way people feel pain (Lea et al., 2011). Results from this type of study can enable genomics services to plan effective future testing. However, owing to a lack of diverse participants, most GWASs currently include data limited to subjects of European descent, which reduces the applicability of findings to populations of non-European origin (Whitley, 2020).

Research of this type has offered some insight into the causes of Crohn's disease. Many genetic and environmental factors are thought to contribute to the development of this inflammatory bowel disorder and an inheritance pattern is not clear; however, Crohn's disease does tend to occur within families and about 15% of people who have Crohn's have a first-degree relative who also has it. A recent GWAS analysing genomic data from over 30,000 people with Crohn's and comparing it with a control group from the general population could implicate specific genes associated with the condition, which could lead to improved predictive abilities. Research data have helped to form better knowledge relating to inflammatory bowel disease and will contribute to advances in clinical management (Sazonovs et al., 2022).

Genomics and nursing

Completion of the Human Genome Project in 2003 initiated a genomics revolution (National Human Genome Research Institute, 2024). In the past 20 years, genomic sequencing has gradually become affordable and accessible. The arrival of next-generation sequencing in 2006 inspired a wave of new methods and applications which revolutionised DNA sequencing (Whitley et al., 2020). Owing to the rapid development of new technologies and their integration into care, all nurses will need to understand basic cell biology and how genetics and genomics determine health. They will need to know how information from the genome can help to improve outcomes and as trusted health professionals they can apply this knowledge to practice, benefitting their local communities (Calzone et al., 2010).

Most nurses have extensive patient contact and are well positioned to increase the uptake of genomic screening to improve outcomes for the general population. In this way the nursing community is equipped with the potential to 'avert adult-onset disorders', including some types of cancer and the associated harms, including early death (Buaki-Sogo and Percival, 2022; Calzone et al., 2010, p.27).

The recognition of the foundations of many common conditions such as cancer, heart disease and diabetes to be both hereditary and non-hereditary in nature means that all nurses, independent of specialty or clinical setting, must have or acquire sufficient knowledge of genetics and genomics to take a family history, identify risk, give information, promote health and refer patients to appropriate services when necessary (Lopes-Júnior et al., 2022). People present at mainstream services with symptoms, health problems or questions before being directed to specialist care, and nurses in these settings must be able to meet their needs. For example, genomic testing may be indicated for those suspected of having a particular condition and referral to specialist services may lead to a diagnosis or to further diagnostic tests, for example, ultrasound scans if polycystic kidney disease is suspected (Lea et al., 2011). If people express concerns about a condition within their family, for example a cardiac condition, families can also be linked with appropriate professionals and services, including genetic counselling, and predictive or pre-symptomatic testing may provide vital information (Lea et al., 2011; Greco and Salveson, 2009). In addition to support around identification of risk and referral for tests, nurses will also provide ongoing support following a diagnosis. Genomics within the nursing role is explored in greater detail in Chapters 3 and 4.

Current pre-treatment screening tests are part of some care pathways and nurses with an awareness of the utility of pharmacogenomics and how information from the genome can inform medicines safety can also improve health outcomes. Pharmacogenomics is explored further in Chapter 7. As more different types of tests become more widely available, nurses can help integrate genomic testing into the service within which they work to improve care in line with newest technologies (Buaki-Sogo and Percival, 2022).

Nurses with an understanding of the NHS genomics infrastructure and some basic knowledge regarding technologies and tests can provide accurate information about genomic testing (Calzone et al., 2010). This includes the ability to ascertain which tests are available and the eligibility criteria to test. The UK Genomic Medicine Service is described in Chapter 2. Nursing skills for accessing current, evidence-based information for patients are essential in any area of care to underpin informed consent for investigations and treatment.

📖 Learning activity

- Visit the British Heart Foundation website. Watch the video and read about different inherited heart conditions.
- Read the section on testing for inherited heart conditions and think about the actions you might take if a patient told you they met one of the listed criteria.
- Follow the link to explore sources of support for people with inherited cardiac conditions.

Inherited heart conditions: https://www.bhf.org.uk/informationsupport/conditions/inherited-heart-conditions

---

Nurses with cultural competence will be aware of the increased incidence and the increased risk of developing some genetic conditions within some patient groups. Some nurses care for those from ethnic population subgroups and can increase local community awareness of genomic risks to health. Genetics and genomics are important in these roles, for example, an awareness that people from Black African, African Caribbean and South Asian (Indian, Pakistani, Bangladeshi) backgrounds are at a higher risk of developing type 2 diabetes at a younger age owing to genetic differences in insulin secretion and fat accumulation (Diabetes UK, 2025).

Health disparities in some groups increase morbidity and mortality resulting from some common conditions. Some cultural customs also increase genetic risks to health, for example consanguinity or cousin marriage is a practice which increases the risk of passing on genetic variants within families. Knowledge regarding health behaviours and understanding the reasons why some groups access health services less than others and do not participate in screening programmes can be useful. It is a nurse's responsibility to try to reduce health inequality created through socio-economic disadvantage in combination with inaccessible services, and addressing observable barriers in systems can facilitate access to care and improve outcomes for all (Matthews Juarez and Juarez, 2011).

A perceived lack of genomics knowledge and confidence within the wider nursing workforce is widely recognised. Many nurses are keen to update their knowledge and develop skills and despite challenges in providing education to the registered workforce, such as budget and time constraints, genomics nursing education is becoming more widely available. As genomics in health care develops, access to appropriate education will empower nurses and enable them to achieve new competencies and to provide the most effective care (Calzone et al., 2018; Daack-Hirsch et al., 2011). Nurses in different roles will have contact with individuals at various stages of their genomics journeys, from the initial identification of risk through to the provision of ongoing care for patients and families. All nurses need some skills including specialist groups such as specialist community public health nurses, health visitors and school nurses. Different aspects of genomics and different nursing skills might be more relevant within some distinct roles, for example child nurses are well placed to identify vulnerable children and introduce safeguarding measures to protect against childhood epigenetic changes.

In genomics, as in other areas of nursing, those working in specialist roles require more advanced skills, for example in relation to requesting tests and reporting results. Specialist skills for nurses in genomics settings are explored in Chapter 4. These nurses are required to identify and manage ethical questions, for example the effects of test results on health insurance, and more information about ethical issues such as legal guidance on managing personal data and ethical guidance on privacy and confidentiality can be found in Chapter 6. People may be prescribed short- or long-term treatments for some genetic and genomic conditions. Gene therapy may also be available for some individuals to restore function and this can be life changing for those with debilitating conditions. In order to care for people effectively, nurses must understand how treatment choices are guided by test results, for example, in the oncology setting precision therapy can be targeted at tumour DNA. Knowledge regarding any drug's intended and any unintended effects can contribute to better management and a better patient experience.

⚕ Nursing genomics skills and knowledge

To integrate genomics effectively onto routine practice, all nurses should be able to:

- Take family histories within the scope of their normal practice and identify genetic and genomic risk factors.
- Access, interpret and give accurate and accessible information about inherited conditions to patients and parents.
- Discuss possible implications of genetic risks for other family members.
- Look at genomic testing criteria in the National Genomic Test Directory.
- Discuss potential testing options and help patients and families make informed choices.
- Refer people to clinical genetics services.
- Support health equality and deliver culturally competent care within their communities.
- Promote health and provide education to reduce the risk of lifestyle and environmental harms.
- Recognise when a person's genetic makeup might affect their response to a medication.
- Advocate for patients and families to facilitate access to genomic services.
- Provide emotional support for patients and families on their genomics journeys.
- Refer to other appropriate support services when indicated, for example in relation to mental health or support at home.
- Seek support to practice safely and effectively.
- Collaborate and coordinate care within a multidisciplinary team.
- Support patients receiving preventive or prophylactic treatment.
- Plan and provide ongoing care for patients and families following a diagnosis.
- Monitor the effectiveness of treatment and identify and help manage adverse drug reactions.

Summary

Clinical practice has evolved to the point at which all nurses need to understand how genomics forms part of holistic assessment and care in terms of eliciting and giving accurate information and appropriate signposting. Genomic medicine can improve outcomes for patients and is something all nurses need to know about. Basic knowledge of the inheritance patterns of common genetic conditions can help nurses to identify genetic risk factors and recognising genomic determinants of health can facilitate effective health promotion and help to prevent disease. The rapid development of genomics technologies and their integration into routine care means that nurses must keep pace with current research and clinical and professional guidance. As the promise of personalised medicine is publicised and patient awareness grows, nurses must develop sufficient genomic literacy to ensure patients benefit from scientific advances.

Genomics educational resources for nurses

- In 2014, Health Education England (now part of NHS England) launched the Genomics Education Programme for health care professionals which can be found at: www.genomicseducation.hee.nhs.uk
- The Road to Genome is a series of podcasts on a range of topics, produced by North East and Yorkshire Genomic Medicine Service. They can be accessed via: Spotify, Amazon Music, Apple Podcasts and Google Podcasts.
- The Your Genome website has multiple accessible resources including animations on the structure of the genome: https://www.yourgenome.org/
- The National Human Genome Research Institute includes resources on the basics of genomics to help improve genomic literacy, including a useful glossary of terms and FAQs for junior and advanced nurses:
  - https://www.genome.gov/About-Genomics/Educational-Resources
  - https://www.genome.gov/genetics-glossary
  - https://www.genome.gov/For-Health-Professionals/Provider-Genomics-Education-Resources/nursing-genomics-faq
- The University of Leicester hosts a Virtual Genetics Education Centre: https://le.ac.uk/vgec
- Behind the Genes is a series of interesting podcasts from Genomics England: https://www.genomicsengland.co.uk/podcasts#:~:text=Introducing%20Behind%20the%20Genes%2C%20previously,take%20you%20behind%20the%20science
- Information about the integration of genomics into UK health care can be found here: https://www.gov.uk/government/publications/genome-uk-the-future-of-healthcare
- Information about UK national genomics testing infrastructure, explored further in the next chapter, can be found here: www.england.nhs.uk/genomics/nhs-genomic-med-service

---

(?) **Quiz – true or false?**

1. To inherit an autosomal dominant genetic condition only one parent must pass on the genetic variant for that condition. True or false?

2. People have 22 pairs of autosomal chromosomes and one pair of sex chromosomes. One from each pair is inherited from their biological mother and one from their biological father. True or false?
3. Only one faulty copy of a gene is needed for a child to inherit an autosomal recessive condition. True or false?
4. Genomics focuses on inheritance patterns for genetic conditions caused by single genes. True or false?
5. Inheriting a pathogenic variant combined with exposure to environmental damage within their lifespan can increase a person's risk of developing some cancers. True or false?

Quiz answers

1. To inherit an autosomal dominant genetic condition only one parent must pass on the genetic variant for that condition. True
2. People have 22 pairs of (somatic?) chromosomes and one pair of sex chromosomes. One from each pair is inherited from their biological mother and one from their biological father. True
3. Only one faulty copy of a gene is needed for a child to inherit an autosomal recessive condition. False
4. Genomics focuses on inheritance patterns for genetic conditions caused by single genes. False
5. Inheriting a pathogenic variant and exposure to environmental damage can increase a person's risk of developing some cancers. True

References

Buaki-Sogo, M. and Percival, N., 2022. Genomic medicine: The role of the nursing workforce. *Nursing Times*, *118*, pp.1–3.

Calzone, K.A., Cashion, A., Feetham, S., Jenkins, J., Prows, C.A., Williams, J.K. and Wung, S.F., 2010. Nurses transforming health care using genetics and genomics. *Nursing Outlook*, *58*(1), pp.26–35.

Calzone, K.A., Kirk, M., Tonkin, E., Badzek, L., Benjamin, C. and Middleton, A., 2018. The global landscape of nursing and genomics. *Journal of Nursing Scholarship*, *50*(3), pp.249–256.

Cancer Research UK, 2023. Genes, DNA and cancer. https://www.cancerresearchuk.org/about-cancer/what-is-cancer/genes-dna-and-cancer (accessed 22 October 2023).

Daack-Hirsch, S., Dieter, V. and Quinn Griffin, M.T., 2011. Integrating genomics into undergraduate nursing education. *Journal of Nursing Scholarship*, *43*(3), pp.223–230.

D'Gama, A.M., Del Rosario, M.C., Bresnahan, M.A., Yu, T.W., Wojcik, M.H. and Agrawal, P.B., 2022. Integrating rapid exome sequencing into NICU clinical care after a pilot research study. *NPJ Genomic Medicine*, *7*(1), p.51.

Diabetes UK, 2025. Ethnicity and Type 2 diabetes. https://www.diabetes.org.uk/about-diabetes/type-2-diabetes/diabetes-ethnicity (accessed 7 March 2025).

Genetic Alliance, 2025. Genetic, rare and undiagnosed conditions explained. https://geneticalliance.org.uk/support-and-information/about-genetics/ (accessed 7 March 2025).

Genomics England, 2024. Generation study. https://www.generationstudy.co.uk/overview-of-the-study (accessed 7 February 2025).

Greco, K.E. and Salveson, C., 2009. Identifying genetics and genomics nursing competencies common among published recommendations. *Journal of Nursing Education*, 48(10), pp.557–565.

Harris, S.E., Riggio, V., Evenden, L., Gilchrist, T., McCafferty, S., Murphy, L., Wrobel, N., Taylor, A.M., Corley, J., Pattie, A. and Cox, S.R., 2017. Age-related gene expression changes, and transcriptome wide association study of physical and cognitive aging traits, in the Lothian Birth Cohort 1936. *Aging (Albany NY)*, 9(12), p.2489.

Harvard University Center on the Developing Child, 2019. Epigenetics and child development: how children's experiences affect their genes. https://developingchild.harvard.edu/resources/what-is-epigenetics-and-how-does-it-relate-to-child-development/ (accessed 7 February 2025).

Horton, R., Wright, C.F., Firth, H.V., Turnbull, C., Lachmann, R., Houlston, R.S. and Lucassen, A., 2024. Challenges of using whole genome sequencing in population newborn screening. *bmj*, *384*, 361.

Hu, M., Cherkaoui, I., Misra, S. and Rutter, G.A., 2020. Functional genomics in pancreatic β cells: recent advances in gene deletion and genome editing technologies for diabetes research. *Frontiers in Endocrinology*, *11*, 576632.

Lea, D.H., Skirton, H., Read, C.Y. and Williams, J.K., 2011. Implications for educating the next generation of nurses on genetics and genomics in the 21st century. *Journal of Nursing Scholarship*, *43*(1), pp.3–12.

Lesk, A.M., 2017. *Introduction to Genomics*. Oxford University Press: Oxford.

Lopes-Júnior, L.C., Bomfim, E. and Flória-Santos, M., 2022. Genetics and genomics teaching in nursing programs in a latin American Country. *Journal of Personalized Medicine*, *12*(7), p.1128.

Matthews-Juarez, P. and Juarez, P.D., 2011. Cultural competency, human genomics, and the elimination of health disparities. *Social Work in Public Health*, *26*(4), pp.349–365.

Mbemi, A., Khanna, S., Njiki, S., Yedjou, C.G. and Tchounwou, P.B., 2020. Impact of gene–environment interactions on cancer development. *International Journal of Environmental Research and Public Health*, *17*(21), p.8089.

National Human Genome Research Institute, 2019. Introduction to genomics. https://www.genome.gov/About-Genomics/Introduction-to-Genomics (accessed 1 August 2023)

National Human Genome Research Institute, 2024. The human genome project. https://www.genome.gov/human-genome-project (accessed 6 March 2025).

NHS England, 2022. Accelerating genomic medicine in the NHS. https://www.england.nhs.uk/long-read/accelerating-genomic-medicine-in-the-nhs/ (accessed 28 August 2024)

NHS England, 2023. The 2023 Genomic Competency Framework for UK nurses. https://www.genomicseducation.hee.nhs.uk/wp-content/uploads/2023/12/2023-Genomic-Competency-Framework-for-UK-Nurses.pdf (accessed 4 December 2023).

NHS, 2021. Turner syndrome. https://www.nhs.uk/conditions/turner-syndrome/ (accessed 28 February 2025).

NMC, 2018 *Standards of Proficiency for Registered Nurses*. NMC: London

Prasad, C., Imrhan, V. and Rew, M., 2011. Introducing nutritional genomics teaching in undergraduate dietetic curricula. *Journal of Nutrigenetics and Nutrigenomics*, *4*(3), pp.165–172.

Richter, J.D. and Zhao, X., 2021. The molecular biology of FMRP: new insights into fragile X syndrome. *Nature Reviews Neuroscience*, *22*(4), pp.209–222.

Sazonovs, A., Stevens, C.R., Venkataraman, G.R., Yuan, K., Avila, B., Abreu, M.T., Ahmad, T., Allez, M., Ananthakrishnan, A.N., Atzmon, G. and Baras, A., 2022. Large-scale sequencing identifies multiple genes and rare variants associated with Crohn's disease susceptibility. *Nature Genetics*, *54*(9), pp.1275–1283.

Shaw, J. and Lurie, I. 2023. Introduction to chromosomes, chromosome disorder outreach. https://chromodisorder.org/introduction-to-chromosomes/ (accessed 31 August 2023).

Smith, H.S., Zettler, B., Genetti, C.A., Hickingbotham, M.R., Coleman, T.F., Lebo, M., Nagy, A., Zouk, H., Mahanta, L., Christensen, K.D. and Pereira, S., 2024. The BabySeq Project: a clinical trial of genome sequencing in a diverse cohort of infants. *The American Journal of Human Genetics*, *111*(10), pp.2094–2106.

Swaroop, A., Chew, E.Y., Bowes Rickman, C. and Abecasis, G.R., 2009. Unraveling a multifactorial late-onset disease: from genetic susceptibility to disease mechanisms for age-related macular degeneration. *Annual Review of Genomics and Human Genetics*, *10*(1), pp.19–43.

Tamimi, A., Serdarevic, D. and Hanania, N.A., 2012. The effects of cigarette smoke on airway inflammation in asthma and COPD: therapeutic implications. *Respiratory Medicine*, *106*(3), pp.319–328.

Tluczek, A., Twal, M.E., Beamer, L.C., Burton, C.W., Darmofal, L., Kracun, M., Zanni, K.L. and Turner, M., 2019. How American nurses association code of ethics informs genetic/genomic nursing. *Nursing Ethics*, *26*(5), pp.1505–1517.

Tonkin, E. and Skirton, H., 2013. The role of genetic/genomic factors in health, illness and care provision. *Nursing Standard*, *28*(12), p.39.

Vancollie, 2021. Genomic surveillance in action. https://www.yourgenome.org/stories/genomic-surveillance-in-action/(accessed 21 August 2023).

Whitley, K.V., Tueller, J.A. and Weber, K.S., 2020. Genomics education in the era of personal genomics: academic, professional, and public considerations. *International Journal of Molecular Sciences*, *21*(3), p.768.

World Health Organization, 2025. Genomics. https://www.who.int/health-topics/genomics#tab=tab_1 (accessed 7 February 2025).

The UK national genomic testing infrastructure

Chapter outline

This chapter provides a brief timeline of the history of genomics in UK health care with reference to significant developments for nursing practice. It provides an overview of current UK infrastructure supporting genetic and genomic testing. Also highlighted are areas of care where genomics makes an important difference, through the types of tests available and the information they can provide, such as pre-natal testing and cancer care.

Introduction

The integration of genomics into routine care can support the identification of an increased risk of developing certain diseases such as cancer and some cardiovascular conditions for a greater number of people. Early identification of risks to health caused by genetic variation can lead to early intervention to improve health outcomes for individuals and families, and nurses in any setting with the ability to assess genomic risk can contribute to improved population health. Pharmacogenomic tests can help predict individual responses to some medicines and the ability to request these tests as part of routine care pathways will contribute to increased medicines safety and efficacy. To realise the benefits of genomic technologies for patients so that information from the genome can be used to inform clinical decision making, the NHS is working towards increasing the availability of tests and the indications for testing (NHS England, 2022). This will mean changes to systems and processes in many practice settings and nurses will be at the heart of many developing services.

An awareness of the care provided by specialist genetics services and knowing how to refer people to these services is an important part of initiating the patient genomics journey. The appropriate skills and knowledge, for example how to determine

DOI: 10.4324/9781003453048-2

whether a patient meets the criteria for a genomic test, how tests are performed and how their results will be reported, enables nurses to provide comprehensive patient information. The UK is the closest it has ever been to the provision of individualised care in NHS services and a long history of the development of genomics precedes this point (Figure 2.1).

Genomic testing in the UK

Specialist genomics health care is provided at mainstream genomics reference centres. In response to the identification of risk or presenting symptoms, patients can be referred to these centres for assessment and genomic testing and to receive treatment and any ongoing support required from multi-disciplinary teams (Buaki-Sogo and Percival, 2022). If a genomic test is indicated and appropriate and a patient meets the eligibility criteria and provides their consent to test, their DNA can be extracted (for example from blood or saliva) to permit detailed examination of their genetic code. Surveying the number and structure of chromosomes or the sequence of the nucleotide base pairs within particular genes can reveal variations to normal patterns and which help to determine a person's health status and can sometimes provide information to support predictions about their future health. Abnormalities identified within the genetic code can contribute to the diagnosis of genetic conditions and help predict individual responses to some medications. Genetic variations can be inherited and may appear in several generations of the same family so some test results can highlight health risks for the presenting or index patient and their close relatives.

The National Genomic Test Directory NGTD (NHS England, 2025) lists all available rare and inherited conditions which can be tested for, with information on who can order them and the patient eligibility criteria for each to ensure that the most appropriate test is requested. The directory is updated regularly so it is best to use the online version: https://www.england.nhs.uk/publication/national-genomic-test-directories/

The purposes of genomic testing include:

- Predictive testing – predictive testing helps to determine the risk of developing a specific genetic disorder for family members of those who have the disorder.
- Diagnostic testing – if a person is suspected to have a genetic disorder, diagnostic testing can confirm whether or not a person has it.
- Pharmacogenomic testing – pharmacogenomic testing is carried out to see how an individual might respond to some medications.
- Reproductive testing – when planning a family, reproductive testing can look for genetic variants carried by biological parents.
- Direct-to-consumer testing – direct-to-consumer testing can be used to find information about an individual's genetic profile and any identifiable risks to their future health from a DNA sample sent by post.
- Forensic testing – forensic testing uses genetic material to identify both suspects and victims of crimes. It is carried out for legal purposes and also helps to identify biological family members. Forensic testing is also used to help identify disaster victims (NHGRI, 2019).

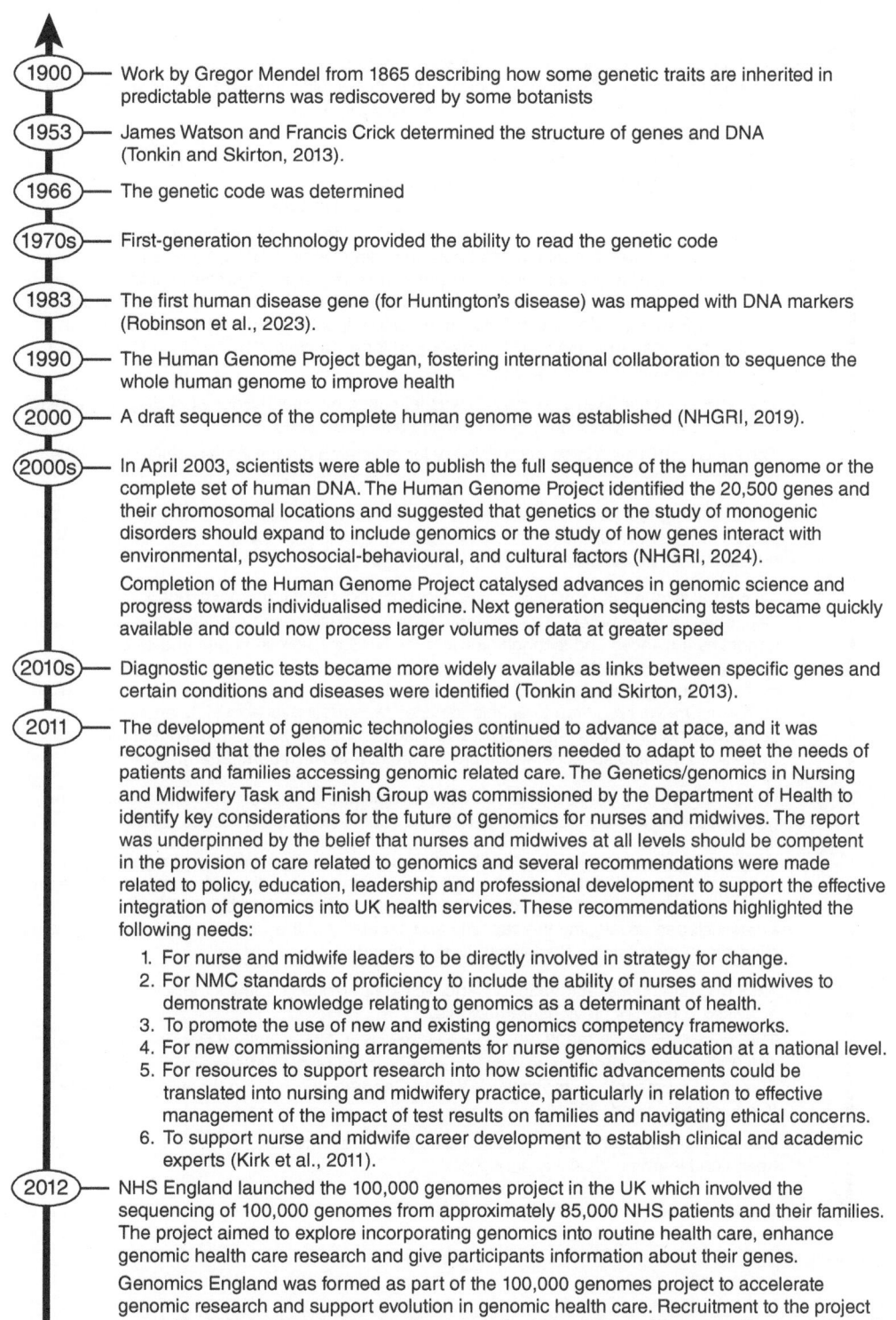

1900 — Work by Gregor Mendel from 1865 describing how some genetic traits are inherited in predictable patterns was rediscovered by some botanists

1953 — James Watson and Francis Crick determined the structure of genes and DNA (Tonkin and Skirton, 2013).

1966 — The genetic code was determined

1970s — First-generation technology provided the ability to read the genetic code

1983 — The first human disease gene (for Huntington's disease) was mapped with DNA markers (Robinson et al., 2023).

1990 — The Human Genome Project began, fostering international collaboration to sequence the whole human genome to improve health

2000 — A draft sequence of the complete human genome was established (NHGRI, 2019).

2000s — In April 2003, scientists were able to publish the full sequence of the human genome or the complete set of human DNA. The Human Genome Project identified the 20,500 genes and their chromosomal locations and suggested that genetics or the study of monogenic disorders should expand to include genomics or the study of how genes interact with environmental, psychosocial-behavioural, and cultural factors (NHGRI, 2024).

Completion of the Human Genome Project catalysed advances in genomic science and progress towards individualised medicine. Next generation sequencing tests became quickly available and could now process larger volumes of data at greater speed

2010s — Diagnostic genetic tests became more widely available as links between specific genes and certain conditions and diseases were identified (Tonkin and Skirton, 2013).

2011 — The development of genomic technologies continued to advance at pace, and it was recognised that the roles of health care practitioners needed to adapt to meet the needs of patients and families accessing genomic related care. The Genetics/genomics in Nursing and Midwifery Task and Finish Group was commissioned by the Department of Health to identify key considerations for the future of genomics for nurses and midwives. The report was underpinned by the belief that nurses and midwives at all levels should be competent in the provision of care related to genomics and several recommendations were made related to policy, education, leadership and professional development to support the effective integration of genomics into UK health services. These recommendations highlighted the following needs:

1. For nurse and midwife leaders to be directly involved in strategy for change.
2. For NMC standards of proficiency to include the ability of nurses and midwives to demonstrate knowledge relating to genomics as a determinant of health.
3. To promote the use of new and existing genomics competency frameworks.
4. For new commissioning arrangements for nurse genomics education at a national level.
5. For resources to support research into how scientific advancements could be translated into nursing and midwifery practice, particularly in relation to effective management of the impact of test results on families and navigating ethical concerns.
6. To support nurse and midwife career development to establish clinical and academic experts (Kirk et al., 2011).

2012 — NHS England launched the 100,000 genomes project in the UK which involved the sequencing of 100,000 genomes from approximately 85,000 NHS patients and their families. The project aimed to explore incorporating genomics into routine health care, enhance genomic health care research and give participants information about their genes.

Genomics England was formed as part of the 100,000 genomes project to accelerate genomic research and support evolution in genomic health care. Recruitment to the project ceased in 2018 but research using the data collected continues (Genomics England, 2025A).

Figure 2.1 The development of genomics for health and care. *(Continued)*

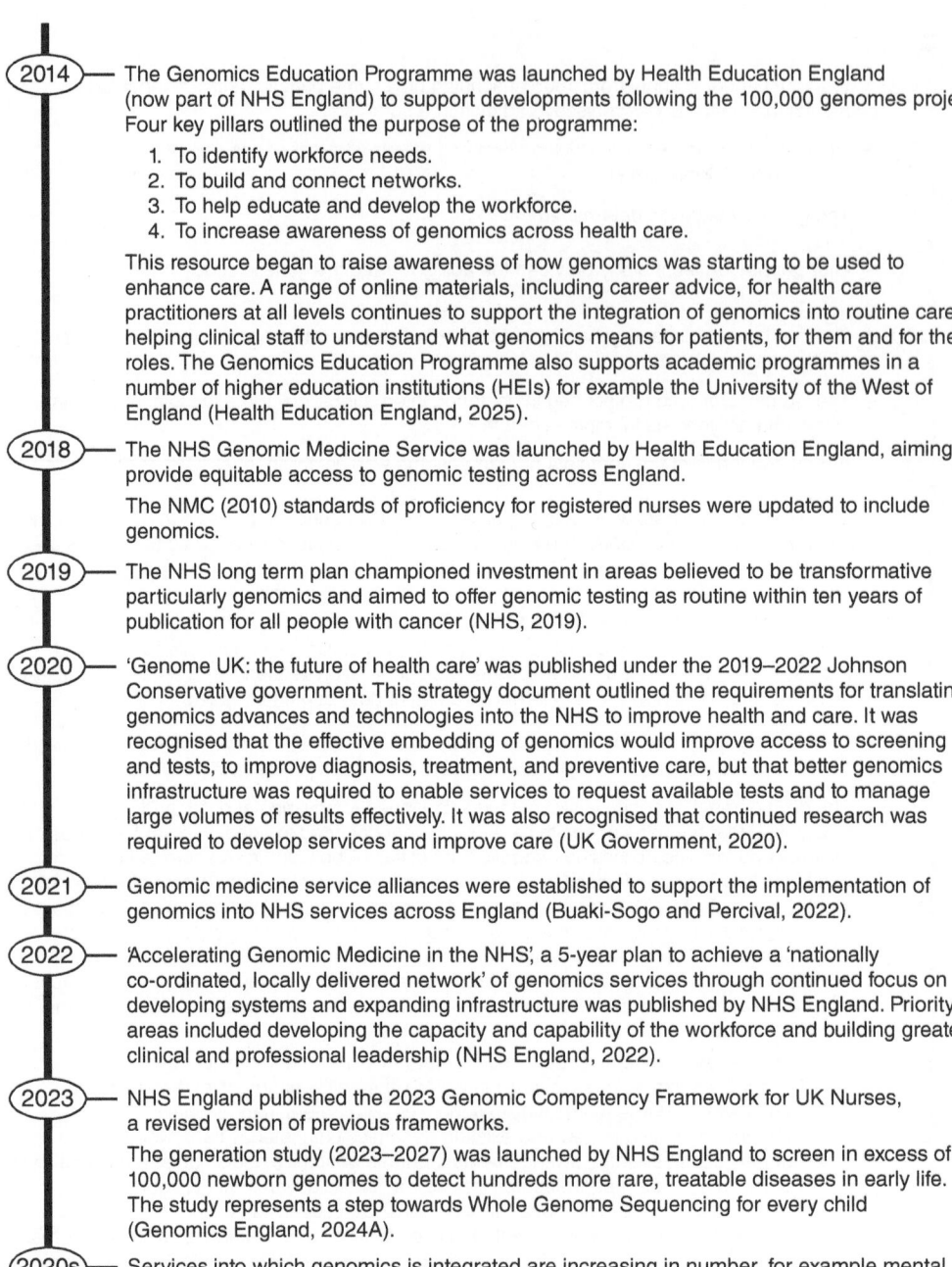

2014 — The Genomics Education Programme was launched by Health Education England (now part of NHS England) to support developments following the 100,000 genomes project. Four key pillars outlined the purpose of the programme:

1. To identify workforce needs.
2. To build and connect networks.
3. To help educate and develop the workforce.
4. To increase awareness of genomics across health care.

This resource began to raise awareness of how genomics was starting to be used to enhance care. A range of online materials, including career advice, for health care practitioners at all levels continues to support the integration of genomics into routine care by helping clinical staff to understand what genomics means for patients, for them and for their roles. The Genomics Education Programme also supports academic programmes in a number of higher education institutions (HEIs) for example the University of the West of England (Health Education England, 2025).

2018 — The NHS Genomic Medicine Service was launched by Health Education England, aiming to provide equitable access to genomic testing across England.

The NMC (2010) standards of proficiency for registered nurses were updated to include genomics.

2019 — The NHS long term plan championed investment in areas believed to be transformative particularly genomics and aimed to offer genomic testing as routine within ten years of publication for all people with cancer (NHS, 2019).

2020 — 'Genome UK: the future of health care' was published under the 2019–2022 Johnson Conservative government. This strategy document outlined the requirements for translating genomics advances and technologies into the NHS to improve health and care. It was recognised that the effective embedding of genomics would improve access to screening and tests, to improve diagnosis, treatment, and preventive care, but that better genomics infrastructure was required to enable services to request available tests and to manage large volumes of results effectively. It was also recognised that continued research was required to develop services and improve care (UK Government, 2020).

2021 — Genomic medicine service alliances were established to support the implementation of genomics into NHS services across England (Buaki-Sogo and Percival, 2022).

2022 — 'Accelerating Genomic Medicine in the NHS', a 5-year plan to achieve a 'nationally co-ordinated, locally delivered network' of genomics services through continued focus on developing systems and expanding infrastructure was published by NHS England. Priority areas included developing the capacity and capability of the workforce and building greater clinical and professional leadership (NHS England, 2022).

2023 — NHS England published the 2023 Genomic Competency Framework for UK Nurses, a revised version of previous frameworks.

The generation study (2023–2027) was launched by NHS England to screen in excess of 100,000 newborn genomes to detect hundreds more rare, treatable diseases in early life. The study represents a step towards Whole Genome Sequencing for every child (Genomics England, 2024A).

2020s — Services into which genomics is integrated are increasing in number, for example mental health and learning disability services.

Figure 2.1 *(Continued)*

Next-generation sequencing was implemented in the 2000s and prompted subsequent focused advances in technology which produced new methods and applications to revolutionise DNA sequencing. The accuracy of DNA sequencing is continually improving and the cost has decreased exponentially since its initial development so it is now affordable and accessible (Whitley et al., 2020). There are now many different ways to read a person's DNA sequences quickly and inexpensively, and powerful computers have been developed to analyse and compare many thousands of sequences concurrently (massive parallel sequencing) (NHGRI, 2025A).

Microarray tests use a high-resolution view of the whole genome to look for abnormalities in the amount of genetic material. These differences can be caused by variations in specific genes (sometimes referred to as mutations) such as the deletion or duplication of particular DNA sequences (Figure 2.2). Single nucleotide polymorphism (SNP) array is a type of microarray which looks at areas of the genome in higher resolution (usually non-coding genes where variation does not affect health but can help to determine patterns of inheritance of genetic variants) containing genes which commonly include differences in base nucleotides, for example the replacement of one base (for example guanine) with a different one (for example adenine). Sequencing tests read DNA sequences and compare them to look for variants. These tests can be requested to look at specific genes or panels of different genes associated with different conditions (Robinson et al., 2024).

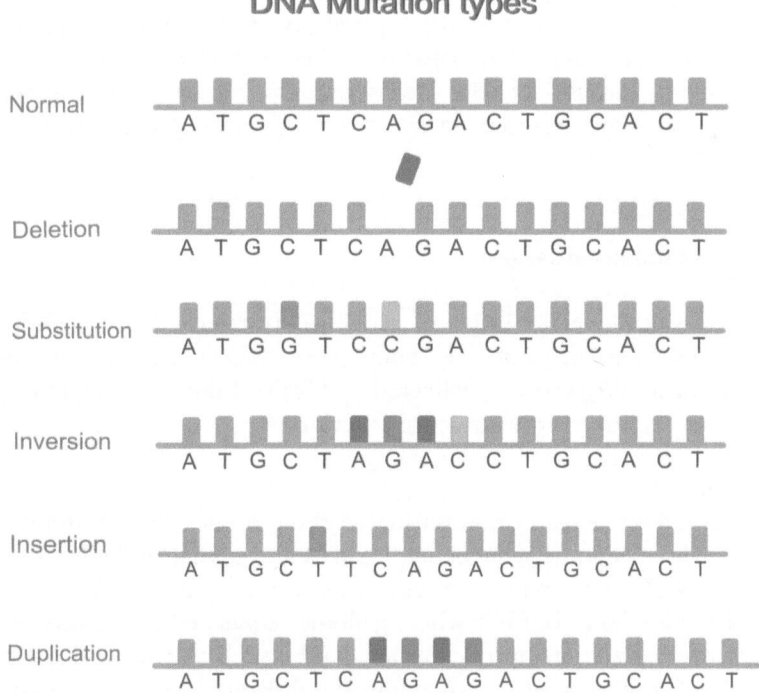

Figure 2.2 Common variations in DNA sequences.

Case study

Joe is 16 and presented at his GP four years ago with weight loss and swollen hands and feet. Urinalysis showed microscopic haematuria and proteinuria, and Joe was referred to a renal consultant who diagnosed him with chronic kidney disease. Joe is on a low sodium and low protein diet but has been attending dialysis for the past year year owing to a sustained decrease in his glomerular filtration rate and increasing haematuria and proteinuria.

This week, Keira, one of the nurses at the renal unit is chatting with Joe's mum who tells her that she has booked an appointment with an audiologist because Joe has been experiencing some loss of hearing. Keira has recently read that some pathogenic gene variants associated with kidney disease can also be responsible symptoms in other body systems, including the ears. She asks to discuss Joe's case with his nephrologist. The nephrologist agrees that Joe meets the testing criteria for test R194 in the NGTD and that a test for a monogenic kidney disorder should be requested.

Joe is anxious about the test because it sounds like it will be invasive, and Keira reassures him that the test can be performed using a blood sample. Joe consents to a referral to the genetic service for genetic counselling. The targeted gene panel test avoids the need for a renal biopsy and in 4 weeks, Joe receives a molecular diagnosis of Alport syndrome, an autosomal recessive disorder. The diagnosis guides a change to Joe's treatment and a monitoring plan to help slow his loss of kidney function and reduce the risk of kidney failure.

Joe's diagnosis has implications for his family members and the genetic counsellor discusses cascade testing for Joe's family with Joe's mum. She also refers Joe to a support group called alport uk (http://www.alportuk.org/).

Keira gathers some information about predictors of monogenic kidney disease and shares it with her colleagues to help enhance nursing practice within the service in relation to considering genetic causes for kidney disease and referring patients for the relevant tests.

This case study was developed using details from Jayasinghe et al. (2021) and Savige and Weinstock (2023).

The NHS genomic medicine service

NHS England

At the time of writing, NHS England provides strategic guidance and support for the integration of genomics into UK health care (Figure 2.3). It commissioned the Genomics Education Programme, delivered by Health Education England (2025), as a self-development resource for health care practitioners.

Genomics England

Genomics England is the lead organisation working on developing and improving the availability of whole genome sequencing. It owns and manages the National Genomic Research Library (NGRL), which stores research data and data from whole genome sequencing. People who have their whole genome sequenced can choose to contribute to future discovery by contributing to data banks such as the NGRL (https://www.genomicsengland.co.uk/patients-participants/data). Researchers can access stored data to explore contributing factors to disease and to support the development of new treatments (Genomics England, 2025B).

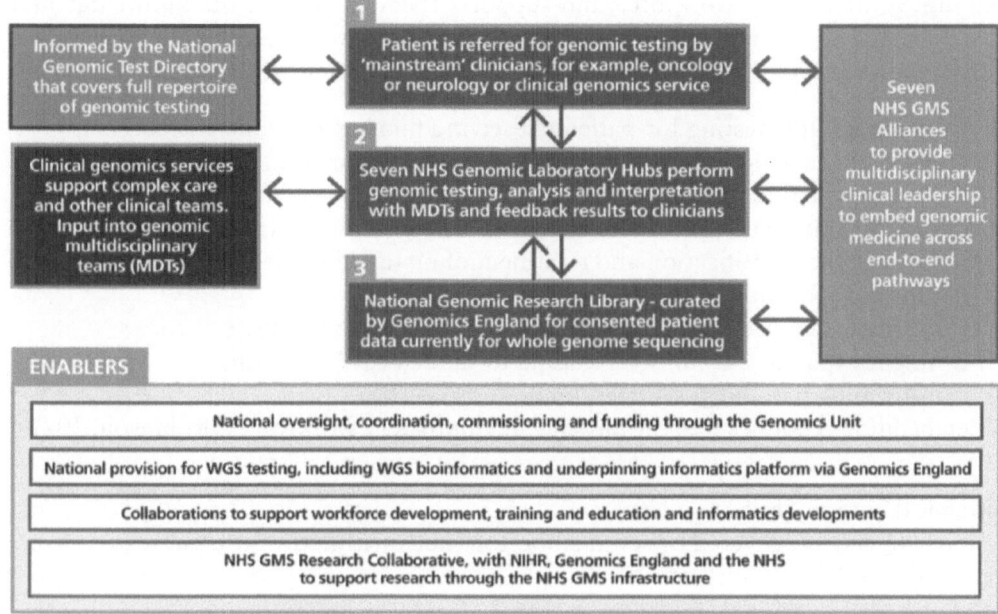

Figure 2.3 Structure of the UK NHS Genomic Medicine Service (NHS England, 2022).

Genomic Medicine Service Alliances

Clinical services across England are supported by seven regional genomic medicine service alliances (GMSAs) (Figure 2.4). The GMSAs are groups of providers who collaborate to embed genomics across regions for local populations. These partnerships work with organisations to support the development of genomics care pathways and nurses are involved in consultations to plan, implement, evaluate and improve these pathways (Buaki-Sogo and Percival, 2022). Responsibilities also include ensuring that each organisation providing genomic medicine has a team that provides education and

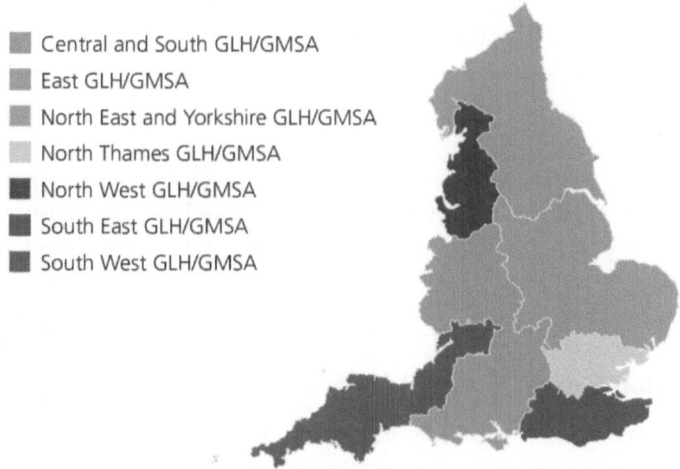

Figure 2.4 The seven genomic medicine service alliances (GMSAs) and genomic laboratory hubs (GLHs) (Health Education England, 2022).

training to the nursing workforce and supports them to acquire the knowledge and skills to support genomic testing and the delivery of care throughout patient genomics journeys. Projects led by the different GMSAs include:

1. Optimising DPD testing for patients receiving fluoropyrimidine chemotherapy – a type of pharmacogenomic test which can use information from the genome to determine whether treatment will be safe for different individuals;
2. embedding familial hypercholesterolaemia services in primary care;
3. improving the identification and treatment of maturity-onset diabetes of the young (a type of monogenic diabetes);
4. delivering a comprehensive service to detect Lynch syndrome;
5. testing for inherited conditions leading to sudden cardiac death;
6. transforming pathology services; and
7. embedding genomics into the nursing and midwifery workforces (Robinson, 2022).

Genomic laboratory hubs
Genomic testing is delivered by seven laboratory hubs within the different regions overseen by the GMSAs.

📖 **Learning activity**

■ Browse the website for each genomic laboratory hub (GLH) and explore the information provided for health care practitioners and patients
  ■ Central and South GLH: https://centralsouthgenomics.nhs.uk/
  ■ East GLH: https://www.eastgenomics.nhs.uk/about-us/genomic-laboratory-hub/
  ■ North East GLH: https://ney-genomics.org.uk/about-genomics/about-the-genomic-medicine-service/genomic-laboratory-hubs/
  ■ North Thames GLH: https://norththamesgenomics.nhs.uk/
  ■ North West GLH: https://mft.nhs.uk/nwglh/
  ■ South East GLH: https://southeastgenomics.nhs.uk/
  ■ South West GLH: https://www.nbt.nhs.uk/south-west-genomic-laboratory-hub

---

Clinical services
The 17 clinical genomics services include national specialist centres and hubs which provide genomics care for patients and families. Care includes risk assessment, genetic counselling, genomic testing and diagnosis, and the clinical management of genetic and genomic conditions.

🔍 **Great Ormond Street Hospital (GOSH)**

Great Ormond Street Hospital (GOSH) is the largest paediatric centre in Europe and a world leader in both genomic research and genomic medicine, including genomic testing leading to targeted interventions before and after birth. Their research teams work closely with

---

patients, parents and the public to understand their needs and take their views into account when developing of genomics services.

GOSH is focusing on the application of genomic technologies to reduce childhood disease including the use of genomic sequencing to accelerate diagnosis and treatment of rare diseases, improving pre-natal diagnosis of genetic conditions and identifying new associations between clinical presentation and genetics.

Recent research includes the use of genomics in improving treatment for childhood diseases such as epilepsy. Epilepsy can be caused by a large number of different genetic variants and international collaboration has shown that rapid genomic sequencing using a standard blood test can improve diagnosis and the appropriate selection of anti-seizure medication in 98% of children.

Further investment into research projects such as this and the management of other rare variants will continue to improve outcomes for individuals and equitability of access to new tests and treatments. (NIHR GOSH, 2025)

National strategy

Key strategy documents outline long-term plans to develop genomic services and increase the availability and accessibility of testing, for example:

- Accelerating Genomic Medicine in the NHS (https://www.england.nhs.uk/publication/accelerating-genomic-medicine-in-the-nhs/) was published by NHS England in 2022. This plan prioritises:
    - the co-creation of services with patients and the public;
    - developing a sustainable genomic testing infrastructure;
    - developing the genomic workforce; and
    - developing national and international genomic collaborations (NHS England, 2022).
- Genome UK (https://www.gov.uk/government/publications/genome-uk-the-future-of-health care) is a strategy paper outlining the vision to extend genomic medicine in the UK. Plans are centred around three key pillars:
    - *diagnosis and personalised medicine* – incorporating genomics advances into routine health care to improve diagnosis, stratification and treatment of illness, with a focus on cancer, rare and inherited disease, pharmacogenomics and infectious disease;
    - *prevention* – enabling predictive and preventative care to improve public health and wellness, with a focus on screening in early life, reconstructive genomic screening and adult screening;
    - *research* – supporting fundamental research and its translation into health services incorporating considerations related to increasing patient participation in research, consent, data management, informatics and genetic diversity (UK Government, 2020).

In 2023, NHS England launched its genomic networks of excellence (NHS England, 2023B). These networks are designed to be partnerships between the NHS academia and industry to combine expertise and resources to inform introduction of new technologies into pathways to increase testing potential and maximise benefits of genomics for patients.

> ## NHS genomic networks of excellence
>
> - Prenatal genomic medicine (https://www.england.nhs.uk/genomics/nhs-genomic-net-works-of-excellence/#prenatal-genomic-medicine).
> - Circulating tumour biomarker testing (https://www.england.nhs.uk/genomics/nhs-genomic-networks-of-excellence/#circulating-tumour-biomarker-testing).
> - Haemato-oncology (https://www.england.nhs.uk/genomics/nhs-genomic-networks-of-excellence/#haemato-oncology).
> - Rare and inherited disease (https://www.england.nhs.uk/genomics/nhs-genomic-networks-of-excellence/#rare-and-inherited-disease).
> - Severe presentation of infectious disease (https://www.england.nhs.uk/genomics/nhs-genomic-networks-of-excellence/#severe-presentation-of-infectious-disease).
> - Improving the identification and outcomes for individuals with inherited and acquired cardiovascular disease (https://www.england.nhs.uk/genomics/nhs-genomic-networks-of-excellence/#cardiovascular-disease).
> - Pharmacogenomic and medicines optimisation (https://www.england.nhs.uk/genomics/nhs-genomic-networks-of-excellence/#pharmacogenomic)
> - Genomics artificial intelligence (https://www.england.nhs.uk/genomics/nhs-genomic-networks-of-excellence/#ai).

Cancer care

Precision oncology is an area that is continuously developing and which well illustrates the proximity of the NHS to delivering on the promise of personalised medicine. For many cancers, clinicians can now select from a range of genomic tests to give them precise information to help treat a particular type of cancer. For example, DNA can be extracted from a patient's cancer cells in samples such as biopsies, blood or bone marrow to compare with DNA from their own cells from blood, saliva or skin samples. This can help oncologists to identify specific mutations leading to the development of tumours and inform treatment choices. Understanding the genetic basis of a person's cancer increases the accuracy of diagnosis and prognosis but may also indicate targeted treatments which can enhance the immune response and act on specific genomic mutations in cancer cell DNA to inhibit cell growth. Furthermore, the ability to obtain genomic data from an individual concerning specific genetic variants which can affect how they can metabolise some cancer drugs helps continue improving the safety of some cancer therapies (Robinson et al., 2024).

Genomic tests can also be used to identify whether a person has a germline (inherited) genetic variant that increases their risk of developing some cancers or a genetic variant causing a cancer pre-disposition syndrome such as Lynch syndrome. Germline variants have implications for individuals and families and may necessitate sharing test results with first-degree relatives and offering them a test for the same variant. This is sometimes referred to as cascade testing. Genomics in cancer care is explored in greater depth in Chapter 5.

> ### :bulb: Reflection point
>
> - Reflect on the range of emotions families waiting for their genomic test results might experience and the skills nurses might use to support patients.
>
> (This learning activity is linked to NHS England (2023A) genomic nursing competency 5.)

Obstetrics and gynaecology

Genomic screening and testing in pregnancy can provide valuable information about the health of unborn babies. This information can help parents know what to expect and inform decisions about the current pregnancy and any future pregnancies. Pre-natal test results can also prepare clinicians to plan for potential interventions.

Pre-natal screening

In the UK, pre-natal screening is offered to all pregnant women to determine the risk of their baby having a number of specific genetic disorders, including chromosomal aneuploidies or conditions caused by differences in the number or structure of chromosomes. Examples include Down syndrome (trisomy 21), Patau syndrome (trisomy 13) and Edwards' syndrome (trisomy 18). These conditions are caused by duplication of part of a chromosome and individuals with these trisomies have three parts making up a specific chromosome instead of two. This extra genetic material creates an increased risk of birth defects and developmental problems (Shaw and Lurie, 2023). Routine pre-natal screening looks for disease-causing variants within the larger population and includes maternal and paternal health histories, a 20-week ultrasound scan and blood tests. This screening is not diagnostic, and any identified anomalies are followed by targeted investigations.

Non-invasive pre-natal testing

If the screening process identifies the increased risk of a foetus having a genetic disorder, a genomic test can be requested to obtain further information from foetal DNA. Nurses can work as part of the multi-disciplinary team to ensure that all women who need them can access pre-natal tests. The NHS England 5-year plan to develop genomics includes consideration of equitable access (NHS England, 2022). Risk factors include a family history or a previous child with a genetic disorder. If siblings or parents are affected by a specific genetic condition and a spontaneous or new (*de novo*) variant is not suspected in a foetus, tests can focus on specific genes, rather than the whole genome (all DNA) or exome (all coding DNA), which can expedite results (Robinson et al., 2024). A maternal age of over 35 increases the risk of chromosomal aneuploidies. Genomic 'red flags' for nurses and midwives also include a positive newborn blood spot test in a previous child, a personal or family history of pregnancy loss, developmental delays in siblings and current or previous genetic investigations for anyone in the family (North East and Yorkshire Genomic Medicine Service, 2024).

DNA from the breakdown of foetal cells including the placenta is released into the bloodstream during pregnancy. This cell-free foetal DNA can be used to test for specific variants which can be detected as early as 6 weeks into pregnancy. Non-invasive pre-natal testing can be performed using a blood sample and is non-invasive compared to traditional tests for foetal chromosomal abnormalities which increase the risk of miscarriage. These tests include chorionic villus sampling from the placenta via the abdomen or cervix and amniocentesis, which involves taking a sample of amniotic fluid. However, if a problem is detected from non-invasive pre-natal testing, further invasive tests may be required to confirm a diagnosis.

Non-invasive pre-natal diagnosis

Non-invasive pre-natal diagnosis can sometimes also be performed using cell-free foetal DNA from maternal blood samples and early diagnosis of a genetic condition can improve the health outcomes of neonates. Diagnostic testing can involve rapid foetal exome screening where next generation sequencing technology is used to detect variants in coding material. This is indicated when multiple anomalies are identified in a foetus, presentation suggests a genetic disorder and molecular diagnosis would guide clinical management.

The R21 test involves targeted testing of coding DNA for at-risk pregnancies and this test is performed to look for a nationally agreed group of conditions. R21 can only be performed using amniotic fluid or chorionic villus samples (Health Education England, 2023).

If a problem is identified in a pre-natal test, samples may then also be taken from the parents' and possibly siblings' plasma to examine their DNA to support a possible diagnosis. The sequencing of SNPs around a gene of interest can help to pinpoint maternal and paternal contributions to foetal genetic variants. A relative haplotype dosage method can be used to detect multiple single gene disorders in a foetus, including Duchenne muscular dystrophy, spinal muscular atrophy and cystic fibrosis when:

- only the baby's father is affected, and the variant can be detected in the mother's plasma DNA (the foetus is positive for the variant);
- the baby's mother and father are both carriers of different autosomal variants and the father's variant is detected in the mother's plasma DNA (the variant comes from foetal DNA);
- neither parent is a carrier of a specific variant identified in a foetus and a spontaneous (*de novo*) variant is suspected (Young et al., 2020).

The suspicion of a sex-linked condition may necessitate determining the sex of an unborn baby to inform management. Duchenne muscular dystrophy in male children is an X-linked recessive condition, which means that it is caused by a gene variant on the X-chromosome. This condition affects males to a greater extent than females because they have only one X-chromosome (the second sex chromosome in males is a Y-chromosome). Female carriers of the condition have a second unaffected X-chromosome to mitigate the issues caused by a genetic fault in the first. Knowing the biological sex of a baby with an X-linked condition can help parents to make decisions about its future. Pre-natal testing and diagnosis can raise some ethical questions as the information obtained may contribute to the decision to terminate a pregnancy. Ongoing research into intrauterine foetal gene editing to correct some congenital conditions, for example some hemoglobinopathies, using the CRISPR-Cas9 complex may also raise ethical questions owing to risks associated with the treatment. This treatment is only used in cases where the risks are balanced by the likelihood of a poor prognosis or a poor quality of life living with a condition for which there are limited treatments (Peddi et al., 2022). Ethical issues in genomic medicine are explored further in Chapter 6.

Newborn screening

Routine screening following birth is a newborn blood spot test (formerly known as the Guthrie 'heel prick' test) which uses a dried blood spot to look for nine conditions including phenylketonuria, thalassaemia, haemophilia and primary haemochromatosis.

📖 Knowledge focus

The Human Genome Project and ethical, social and legal implications

The Human Genome Project involved the collaboration of thousands of scientists from North America, the UK, Japan, France, Germany, China and others over 13 years and culminated in the sequencing of the complete human genome.

The project and the necessary considerations associated with managing the personal data of participants, including their DNA, prompted researchers to realise that obtaining information from the genome could raise some ethical concerns. These include the privacy and confidentiality of genomic information and the potential for discriminatory use of genomic information, for example the effects on health insurance of the disclosure of pathogenic variants, particularly in the US. The psychological impact and stigmatisation related to genetic differences were also recognised as an issue in addition to reproductive questions raised by genomic information and uncertainties for individuals associated with genomic tests and resulting harms such as anxiety.

These concerns prompted the setting up of a programme to explore the ethical, social and legal implications of obtaining and storing information from the genome and the US National Genome Research Institute (NHGRI) continues to fund research into genomic health care to examine ethical legal and social implications which arise as new services develop (NHGRI, 2025B).

Pharmacogenomic testing

An individual's genotype codes for inherited traits caused by normal allelic variation such as eye colour, hair colour and blood type. Some genotypes include variations in the genes which determine how the body will process medicines. This type of variant can influence both the efficacy of and the risk of harm from some medicines. Pharmacogenomic tests are performed to identify specific variations which affect the body's ability to metabolise or break down a drug for elimination. This can expose individuals to adverse drug reactions caused by the accumulation and potentially harmful plasma levels of drug. Assays can be selected which look at variants within a single gene or use microarrays to identify most known variants in a single test (Johnson et al., 2020).

It is becoming normal practice for nurses to request pharmacogenomic tests prior to the prescription or administration of certain drugs where laboratory-based testing is available. For example, NICE has released new guidance (https://www.nice.org.uk/

guidance/dg59) on CYP2C19 genotype testing to assess whether clopidogrel will be a suitable antiplatelet drug for people who have had an ischaemic stroke or a transient ischaemic attack (NICE, 2024). Some 32% of people in the UK have a variant of the CYP2C19 enzyme affecting the metabolism of clopidogrel into its active form and for these individuals a different drug would produce a better effect. Laboratory testing is more cost effective, but point of care testing can be used when laboratory tests are not available in a specific area (Burns, 2023).

Within a given population there will be a range of reactions to any drug and building a database of responses matched with individual genotypes can contribute to the development of individualised prescribing. In addition to improving drug efficacy and patient experience by guiding dosing decisions, pre-treatment pharmacogenomic testing will reduce unnecessary drug use and the costs this creates for health services (Johnson et al., 2020). More information about pharmacogenomics can be found in Chapter 7.

Genomic testing and the nursing role

With the rapid pace of scientific discovery, knowledge about how genomics can be used effectively within health services is expanding and nurses can support the successful integration of genomic medicine into mainstream health care (Buaki-Sogo and Percival, 2022). Awareness of the national testing infrastructure and the roles of the different organisations within can help nurses to signpost or refer patients to appropriate services.

Effective nursing care related to genomics is dependent on specific proficiencies and all nurses should be able to:

- identify patients who may benefit from genomic testing;
- access information about genomic testing pathways and discuss testing with patients; and
- refer patients to specialist services for genetic counselling and genomic testing (Buaki-Sogo and Percival, 2022).

The genomics knowledge and skills required by all nurses is explored further in Chapter 3. Nursing responsibilities span a breadth of care and in addition to acquiring the basic knowledge to enhance their routine practice, many nurses will be concerned with reviewing the services within which they work to explore how processes might be adapted to include consideration of genomic risk and links to genomic testing services where appropriate. The design of health care policies related to genomics can only be effective if it includes the perspectives of nurses and nursing organisations because some nurses will be pivotal in the integration of genomics across UK health services in line with new research and scientific advances (Calzone et al., 2010).

As genomic medicine develops, some nurses will have the opportunity to help define how genomic testing is integrated into practice within their areas or to improve processes within care settings where genomic testing and targeted treatment are already integrated (Buaki-Sogo and Percival, 2022). This may involve the planning and coordination of new elements of care, and/or the evaluation of services and any necessary improvement. Nurses have the ability to advocate for groups who would benefit from improved access to care and their unique perspectives will help providers to consider local populations and to support access to effective care for all. In addition to their clinical skills, nurses leading in establishing and running services effectively require the skills and knowledge for improvement and innovation within health settings.

Genetic Alliance UK

Some organisations provide valuable information for health care professionals and patients. Genetic Alliance UK (https://geneticalliance.org.uk/) is a network of organisations supporting people with genetic and undiagnosed conditions in the UK. Their website hosts extensive information for individuals and organisations about living with genetic conditions. This website also contains links to sources of support for those in need.

Genetic Alliance UK lead two longstanding groups you may wish to read about:

- Rare disease UK: https://www.raredisease.org.uk/
- Swan UK: https://geneticalliance.org.uk/support-and-information/swan-uk-syndromes-without-a-name/

Research and nursing practice

The current Royal College of Nursing (RCN) definition of nursing includes working within organisations to provide specialised and complex interventions as a recognised component of the nursing role (RCN, 2024). Some nurses work within specialist genomics roles and both administer and monitor the effects of newly developed treatments. For new drugs, nurses must understand the mode of action and feel confident to discuss this information with patients so that they can provide informed consent. Understanding any associated risks can also inform discussion with patients and help nurses to predict and to mitigate potential harm through effective monitoring. New treatments are subject to post-marketing surveillance and are recognised by the black triangle symbol in the British National Formulary. The submission of yellow card data relating to adverse drug reactions caused by new or 'black triangle' drugs by nurses contributes to increased patient safety (MHRA, 2014).

For example, novel therapies are being developed to simulate the body's own repair mechanisms and help tissue regenerate following a myocardial infarction (heart attack). During a myocardial infarction, cardiac tissue can be deprived of oxygen, causing the death of some heart muscle cells. Current research into regenerative treatment is exploring the use of mRNA, or modified messenger RNA therapy to regenerate damaged myocardium. Modified mRNA can also be used to grow transplant tissues to replace damaged heart tissue. As such therapies are introduced into practice, nurses working in cardiac rehabilitation will be required to measure the effectiveness of medicines and to determine the optimal dose and timing of administration and conditions for optimal use and record side effects to help construct an accurate safety profile for future use (Bois et al., 2025).

Nurses can facilitate patient enrolment in research projects for new treatments or for other aspects of genomic medicine where appropriate and patient data comprise an essential and valuable part of scientific discovery. Many patients are happy to consent to their data being shared and to contribute to clinical advances in genomic testing and related care. But within any research project, it is important that patients are given the opportunity to voice what matters to them and to be able to speak about their experiences, and for their views to be acknowledged (Hastings Ward et al., 2022). Our Future Health is a large-scale UK health research programme that aims to explore the genetic and genomic basis of population health. The findings from this study will enable new ways of detecting and measuring risk and treating and preventing disease. Our Future Health is a charity working in partnership with the NHS. People can read more about the study, enrol online and go to a local clinic if they wish to give a DNA (blood) sample (Our Future Health, 2025). Nurses who promote this study and other research projects can raise awareness about the benefits of genomics and increase the amount of available data for researchers.

📖 Knowledge focus

The Deciphering Developmental Disorders study

The Deciphering Developmental Disorders study was launched in 2011, and the results were published in 2023. This study was focused on the genomic diagnosis of rare paediatric disease in the UK and Ireland. A total of 13,610 participants were involved, 9859 of whom were enrolled with parents who were also willing to have their DNA tested.

Consultant clinical geneticists sought to recruit parents whose children had:

- neurodevelopmental disorders
- congenital anomalies
- abnormal growth measurements
- dysmorphic features
- unusual behavioural phenotypes
- severe undiagnosed genetic disorders.

Genomic tests, including exome screening and SNP genotyping of family DNA, were performed to look for pathogenic genetic variants that could be contributing to the child's presentation.

A total of 4484 participants received a diagnosis, 3599 of whom were enrolled as parent/child trios.

The molecular diagnoses achieved will provide lifelong benefits for children with severe monogenic developmental disorders and their families. About 60 new disorders were discovered and data from the study contributed to our growing knowledge about the origins of disease and to future genomic health research (Wright et al., 2023).

Genomics, bacteria and viruses

In addition to the human organism, genomic science is advancing the study of microorganisms with which the human genome interacts, including pathogens such as bacteria and viruses. The use of new technologies to explore these interactions can provide opportunities to develop new approaches to the prevention and management of disease, for example, protection against the influenza virus (World Health Organization, 2020). Vaccinations given by nurses and health visitors, for example in early childhood, help the immune system to recognise pathogens. Studying the genomics of viruses supports genetic engineering, which helps develop vaccines for viruses such as hepatitis B, whooping cough and some strains of meningitis (Lesk, 2017). *Helicobacter pylori* is a bacterium usually contracted during childhood that infects the stomach of half of the global population, and genomic screening can determine whether a patient has a strain of *H. pylori* likely to be the cause of clinical issues such as gastritis, gastrointestinal ulcers and some cancers (Lesk, 2017).

The early twenty-first century has demonstrated how quickly infectious diseases can spread, including AIDS, SARS, H5N1 and Zika viruses. Nurses have a duty to understand the global disease burden and the health implications of migration, travel and displacement (Tluczek et al., 2019). Genomics has a role to play in public health care related to bacterial and viral infections and surveillance and managing outbreaks (World Health Organization, 2020). Whole genome sequencing can help identify different strains of tuberculosis. Other viruses under continued surveillance include ebola in Africa, a deadly virus from which 90% of those infected die within days.

On a smaller scale, scientists have the ability to sequence bacterial DNA to manage outbreaks within organisations of infections including *Clostridioides difficile* and methicillin-resistant *Staphylococcus aureus* (MRSA), and to decolonise individual staff members to prevent transmission and further outbreaks (Eyre, 2022). Genomic screening of bacteria such as *Escherichia coli* can help to control outbreaks because determining how new cases are related to those already sequenced can identify transmission patterns and prevent spread (Lesk, 2017).

Genomics technologies can help scientists to understand routes of transmission and to help limit the spread of severe respiratory viruses. Genomics was important in managing Covid-19 and researchers could quickly sequence the virus's genetic material and use its modified mRNA to create a vaccine (Gunadi et al., 2021). Genetic information including that from participants in previous genome wide association studies and those buying private or direct to consumer tests was used to help identify individuals at increased risk of suffering with more severe symptoms from the virus (Covid-19 Host Genetics Initiative, 2021). Following the Covid-19 pandemic, the tracking of variants of the virus is conducted through sequencing the viral genome. Genomic scientists can identify whether previous vaccines administered will protect the population against new variants. In this way, genomic data informs policy, strategy and health care planning to safeguard public health.

In 2024, the UK health security agency published a 5-year pathogen genomics strategy to help us better use genomic technology to:

- identify the source of pathogen outbreaks;
- track transmission of disease;
- understand the human immune response to a pathogens;
- develop effective vaccines; and
- determine optimal treatments and detect antimicrobial resistance (UK Government, 2024).

Genomics and anti-microbial resistance

In 2024, a new 5-year plan was published to tackle antimicrobial resistance which included the development of new surveillance systems to measure, understand and predict how resistant pathogens spread (UK Government, 2024). Antimicrobial resistance is a global problem, and current research is focused on screening the genomes of microbes to study the genes associated with resistance and to support the prediction and prevention of resistance to commonly used drugs (World Health Organization, 2020). Extensive genomic research into the development of antibiotic resistance in bacteria such as *Staphylococcus aureus* has contributed to hospital infection prevention and control guidelines (Lesk, 2017). Avoiding the transmission of MRSA is a significant part of the nursing role in many settings and can contribute to the prevention health care-acquired infections, which cause significant harm and increase hospital stays for some patients.

Nurse must also assist in protecting antibiotics for future generations by avoiding inappropriate use. Research into developing diagnostic tests that can rapidly identify specific pathogens and sensitivities can support the prescription of narrow spectrum antimicrobials. Areas within which patient tests are close to being available include pneumonia in secondary care, sepsis and sexually transmitted infections in primary care. Nurses will soon be able to perform these tests widely to support antimicrobial stewardship (Johnson et al., 2020).

 Skills focus

Standard infection control precautions to prevent the transmission of microorganisms and pathogens

Standard infection control precautions (SICPs) are to be used by all staff, in all care settings, at all times, for all patients whether infection is known to be present or not, to ensure the safety of those being cared for, staff and visitors in the care environment.

There are 10 elements of SICPs:

1. patient placement/assessment of infection risk;
2. hand hygiene;
3. respiratory and cough hygiene;
4. personal protective equipment;
5. safe management of the care environment;
6. safe management of care equipment;
7. safe management of health care linen;
8. safe management of blood and body fluids;
9. safe disposal of waste (including sharps); and
10. occupational safety/managing prevention of exposure (including sharps).

From the National Infection Prevention and Control Manual for England (NHS England, 2024): https://www.england.nhs.uk/national-infection-prevention-and-control-manual-nipcm-for-england/chapter-1-standard-infection-control-precautions-sicps/

📖 Learning activity

- Think about how you might explain both anti-microbial resistance and anti-microbial stewardship to a patient.
- Read some key guidance for anti-microbial stewardship and consider the parts of your practice which this guidance most applies to.

Antimicrobial stewardship: https://bnf.nice.org.uk/medicines-guidance/antimicrobial-stewardship/

Summary

All nurses require knowledge of the UK national genomics testing infrastructure to be able to facilitate access to genomic tests for those who need them. Nurses in all settings can evaluate the services within which they work to determine whether there are effective mechanisms in place to help staff to consider genomic testing for those who may benefit and to discuss this option with them. Having an awareness of current health research is an important part of the nursing role and nurses should have a basic understanding of the trajectory of scientific progress in genomics. This will enable them to predict how forthcoming changes might affect their role and to access information and education, for example the Genomics Education Programme, to enhance both knowledge and patient care.

Learn more

- The Royal College of Obstetricians and Gynaecologists has produced some podcasts to support health care professionals to gain insight into the use of genomic medicine in obstetrics and gynaecology: https://www.rcog.org.uk/about-us/quality-improvement-clinical-audit-and-research-projects/genomics-at-rcog/genomics-resources-and-learning-plan/rcog-genomics-podcasts-genomics-in-the-subspecialties-of-obstetrics-gynaecology/
- The UK Health Security Agency data dashboard shows the public health data for example on respiratory viruses, health care-associated infections and antimicrobial stewardship, which informs public health decision making: https://ukhsa-dashboard.data.gov.uk/
- This interesting NHGRI news article reports on managing the spread of pathogens in nursing homes: https://www.genome.gov/news/news-release/multidrug-resistant-pathogens-living-on-the-skin-spread-widely-in-nursing-homes
- The Genomics Education Programme Knowledge Hub contains information on the clinical application of Whole Genome Sequencing: https://www.genomicseducation.hee.nhs.uk/genotes/knowledge-hub/whole-genome-sequencing/
- This RCN article contains information about genomic testing within nursing practice: https://www.rcn.org.uk/magazines/Clinical/2022/Jun/Genomics-DNA-inherited-risk-and-your-patients-family-tree

Information for patients and the public

- The NHS website contains accessible information for patients about genomic testing: https://www.nhs.uk/conditions/genetic-and-genomic-testing/

References

Bois, A., Grandela, C., Gallant, J., Mummery, C. and Menasché, P., 2025. Revitalizing the heart: strategies and tools for cardiomyocyte regeneration post-myocardial infarction. *npj Regenerative Medicine*, *10*(1), p.6.

Buaki-Sogo, M. and Percival, N., 2022. Genomic medicine: the role of the nursing workforce. *Nursing Times*, *118*, pp.1–3.

Burns, 2023. NICE to recommend genetic testing before prescribing clopidogrel. *The Pharmaceutical Journal*. https://pharmaceutical-journal.com/article/news/nice-to-recommend-genetic-testing-before-prescribing-clopidogrel (accessed 5 March 2025).

Calzone, K.A., Cashion, A., Feetham, S., Jenkins, J., Prows, C.A., Williams, J.K. and Wung, S.F., 2010. Nurses transforming health care using genetics and genomics. *Nursing Outlook*, *58*(1), pp.26–35.

COVID-19 Host Genetics Initiative, 2021. Mapping the human genetic architecture of COVID-19. *Nature*, *600*, 472–477. https://doi.org/10.1038/s41586-021-03767-x

Eyre, D.W., 2022. Infection prevention and control insights from a decade of pathogen whole-genome sequencing. *Journal of Hospital Infection*, *122*, pp.180–186.

Genomics England, 2024. Generation study. https://www.generationstudy.co.uk/overview-of-the-study (accessed 7 February 2025).

Genomics England, 2025A. 100,000 Genome Project. https://www.genomicsengland.co.uk/initiatives/100000-genomes-project (accessed 11 March 2025).

Genomics England, 2025B. How your data is used. https://www.genomicsengland.co.uk/patients-participants/data (accessed 11 March 2025).

Gunadi, Wibawa, H., Hakim, M.S., Marcellus, Trisnawati, I., Khair, R.E., Triasih, R., Irene, Afiahayati, Iskandar, K. and Siswanto, 2021. Molecular epidemiology of SARS-CoV-2 isolated from COVID-19 family clusters. *BMC Medical Genomics*, *14*, pp.1–14.

Hastings Ward, J., Middleton, R., McCormick, D., White, H., Kherroubi Garcia, I., Simmonds, S., Chandramouli, L. and Hart, A., 2022. Research participants: critical friends, agents for change. *European Journal of Human Genetics*, *30*(12), pp.1309–1313.

Health Education England, 2025. Genomics Education Programme, Genomic Laboratory hubs. https://www.genomicseducation.hee.nhs.uk/genotes/knowledge-hub/genomic-laboratory-hubs/ (accessed 4 March 2025).

Health Education England, 2023. R21: Rapid pre-natal exome sequencing. https://www.genomicseducation.hee.nhs.uk/genotes/knowledge-hub/r21-rapid-prenatal-exome-sequencing/ (accessed 11 March 2025).

Health Education England, 2025. Genomics Education Programme. https://www.genomicseducation.hee.nhs.uk/about-us/ (accessed 8 March 2025).

Jayasinghe, K., Stark, Z., Kerr, P.G., Gaff, C., Martyn, M., Whitlam, J., Creighton, B., Donaldson, E., Hunter, M., Jarmolowicz, A. and Johnstone, L., 2021. Clinical impact of genomic testing in patients with suspected monogenic kidney disease. *Genetics in Medicine*, *23*(1), pp.183–191.

Johnson, E., Janus, J., Blackburn, L., Kroese, M. and Babb de Villiers, C., 2020. *Genomic Innovation: Technologies for Personalised Medicine. The AHSN Network*.

Kirk, M., Campalani, S., Doris, F., Heron, J., Mannion, G., Metcalfe, A., Patch, C., Permalloo, N., Shepherd, M. and Calzone, K.,2011. Genetics/genomics in nursing and midwifery: Task and Finish Group report to the nursing and midwifery professional advisory board.

Lesk, A.M., 2017. *Introduction to Genomics*. Oxford University Press: Oxford.

MHRA, 2014. The black triangle scheme. https://www.gov.uk/drug-safety-update/the-black-triangle-scheme-or (accessed 17 March 2025).

North East and Yorkshire Genomic Medicine Service, 2024. Genomic red flags. https://ney-genomics.org.uk/wp-content/uploads/2024/07/A5_folded.pdf (accessed 7 March 2025).

NHGRI, 2019. Introduction to genomics. https://www.genome.gov/About-Genomics/Introduction-to-Genomics (accessed 16 August 2023).

NHGRI, 2024. The human genome project. https://www.genome.gov/human-genome-project (accessed 6 March 2025).

NHGRI, 2025A. Technology advances since the human genome project. https://www.genome.gov/dna-day/15-ways/dna-sequencing (accessed 4 March 2025).

NHGRI, 2025B. Ethical, legal and social implications research program. https://www.genome.gov/Funded-Programs-Projects/ELSI-Research-Program-ethical-legal-social-implications (accessed 20 March 2025).

NHS, 2019. The NHS Long term plan. https://www.longtermplan.nhs.uk/ (accessed 11 March 2025).

NHS England, 2022. Accelerating genomic medicine in the NHS. https://www.england.nhs.uk/long-read/accelerating-genomic-medicine-in-the-nhs/ (accessed 28 August 2024).

NHS England, 2023A. The 2023 Genomic Competency Framework for UK Nurses. https://www.genomicseducation.hee.nhs.uk/wp-content/uploads/2023/12/2023-Genomic-Competency-Framework-for-UK-Nurses.pdf (accessed 28 May 2025).

NHS England, 2023B. Genomic Networks of Excellence. https://www.england.nhs.uk/genomics/nhs-genomic-networks-of-excellence/ (accessed 7 March 2025).

NHS England, 2024. National Infection Prevention and Control Manual (NIPCM) for England. https://www.england.nhs.uk/national-infection-prevention-and-control-manual-nipcm-for-england/ (accessed 6 March 2025).NHS England, 2025. National genomic test directory. https://www.england.nhs.uk/publication/national-genomic-test-directories/ (accessed 28 May 2025).

NICE, 2024. CYP2C19 genotype testing to guide clopidogrel use after ischaemic stroke or transient ischaemic attack. https://www.nice.org.uk/guidance/dg59 (accessed 6 March 2025).

NIHR GOSH, 2025. https://www.gosh.nhs.uk/our-research/our-research-infrastructure/nihr-great-ormond-street-hospital-brc/about-our-biomedical-research-centre/our-research-themes/genomic-medicine/ (accessed 12 March 2025).

NMC (2010) *Standards for competence for registered nurses*. NMC, London. https://www.nmc.org.uk/globalassets/sitedocuments/standards/nmc-standards-for-competence-for-registered-nurses.pdf

Our Future Health, 2025. https://ourfuturehealth.org.uk/ (accessed 28 May 2025).

Peddi, N.C., Ramesh, H.M., Gude, S.S., Gude, S.S. and Vuppalapati, S., 2022. Intrauterine fetal gene therapy: is that the future and is that future now? *Cureus*, 14(2).

RCN, 2024. Definition and principles of nursing. https://www.rcn.org.uk/Professional-Development/Definition-and-principles-of-nursing (accessed 6 March 2025).

Robinson, J., 2022. Everything you need to know about the NHS genomic medicine service. https://pharmaceutical-journal.com/article/feature/everything-you-need-to-know-about-the-nhs-genomic-medicine-service (accessed 11 March 2025).

Robinson, S.L., Seneviratne, N. and Dandapani, M., 2024. Understanding recent advances in genomic testing in paediatric oncology. *Paediatrics and Child Health*.

Savige, J. and Weinstock, B.A., 2023. What patients want to know about genetic testing for kidney disease. *Frontiers in Medicine*, 10, p.1201712.

Shaw, J. and Lurie, I., 2023 Introduction to chromosomes, chromosome disorder outreach. https://chromodisorder.org/introduction-to-chromosomes/ (accessed 31 August 2023).

Tluczek, A., Twal, M.E., Beamer, L.C., Burton, C.W., Darmofal, L., Kracun, M., Zanni, K.L. and Turner, M., 2019. How American nurses association code of ethics informs genetic/genomic nursing. *Nursing Ethics*, 26(5), pp.1505–1517.

Tonkin, E. and Skirton, H., 2013. The role of genetic/genomic factors in health, illness and care provision. *Nursing Standard (through 2013)*, 28(12), p.39.

UK Government, 2020. Genome UK: the future of healthcare. https://www.gov.uk/government/publications/genome-uk-the-future-of-healthcare (accessed 28 August 2024).

UK Government, 2024. Confronting antimicrobial resistance 2024–2029. https://www.gov.uk/government/publications/uk-5-year-action-plan-for-antimicrobial-resistance-2024-to-2029/confronting-antimicrobial-resistance-2024-to-2029 (accessed 6 March 2025).

Whitley, K.V., Tueller, J.A. and Weber, K.S., 2020. Genomics education in the era of personal genomics: academic, professional, and public considerations. *International Journal of Molecular Sciences*, 21(3), p.768.

World Health Organization, 2020. GLASS whole-genome sequencing for surveillance of antimicrobial resistance. https://iris.who.int/bitstream/handle/10665/334354/9789240011007-eng.pdf?sequence=1 (accessed 5 March 2025).

Wright, C.F., Campbell, P., Eberhardt, R.Y., Aitken, S., Perrett, D., Brent, S., Danecek, P., Gardner, E.J., Chundru, V.K., Lindsay, S.J. and Andrews, K., 2023. Genomic diagnosis of rare pediatric disease in the United Kingdom and Ireland. *New England Journal of Medicine*, 388(17), pp.1559–1571.

Young, E., Bowns, B., Gerrish, A., Parks, M., Court, S., Clokie, S., Mashayamombe-Wolfgarten, C., Hewitt, J., Williams, D., Cole, T. and Allen, S., 2020. Clinical service delivery of noninvasive prenatal diagnosis by relative haplotype dosage for single-gene disorders. *The Journal of Molecular Diagnostics*, 22(9), pp.1151–1161.

Genomics knowledge and skills for all nurses

Chapter outline

Progress in genomic medicine is influencing changes to the design and delivery of UK health services and the roles of the nurses who staff them. As clinical services incorporate new genomic research findings and technologies into the care they provide, nurses in all areas of practice will require the skills and knowledge to discuss genomics with patients. This chapter outlines why it is important that all nurses develop knowledge about genomic contributions to health and can identify risk factors. Fluency in basic biosciences, including an understanding of pathogenic genetic variation and inheritance patterns for common conditions, is an essential element of this understanding. Nurses must also appreciate the relationship between genetic risk and environmental and lifestyle factors in order to educate patients about risk and to promote health effectively. Familiarity with national screening and early prevention programmes and with the national genomic testing infrastructure facilitates the timely signposting of people who need it to appropriate services.

Introduction

Progress in genomic medicine has precipitated an increase in the accessibility and use of genomic technology and genomics now underpins all aspects of health care and affects all health professionals (Calzone et al., 2010). The extension of genomics care beyond clinical genetics services to integration into many other aspects of care, for example the prevention and management of common chronic conditions such as heart disease and type 2 diabetes, means that health care practitioners need to develop new skills and knowledge required for their roles (Campion et al., 2019). It has long been recognised that nurses need to have knowledge of genetics and genomics in health care regardless of where they work (Tonkin and Skirton, 2013) and in 2022, NHS England outlined plans for 'upskilling' the workforce and developing genomics capability. The focus of

DOI: 10.4324/9781003453048-3

these plans was the provision of education at all levels from formal training for genetic scientists, masters' programmes for clinical staff through to opportunities for the general raising of genomics awareness (NHS England, 2022).

Research into nursing competence in genomics has considered the needs of patients at each stage of their journey and what all nurses need to know to meet those needs (Kirk et al., 2014). In all fields of practice, nurses must be equipped with basic genetics knowledge encompassing common genetic conditions and their inheritance patterns, and epigenetic changes across the lifespan and their effects on gene expression. This will help them to recognise an increased risk of disease for individuals, families and community groups and to meet their responsibility to recognise those who would benefit from genomic services owing to increased risks to health brought about by their ethnic ancestry, family health history, lifestyle or additional socio-cultural factors (Greco and Salveson, 2009). Following the identification of risk, familiarity with national screening programmes and other genomic services helps nurses to direct patients to the services and professionals they need.

Increased public interest in the concept of personalised medicine means that patients are initiating conversations within which nurses must feel confident to answer questions accurately regarding genomic testing and targeted treatments (Buaki-Sogo and Percival, 2022). An understanding of how genomic science can improve health outcomes and the utility of new technologies is also required in preparation to support patients and families effectively (Tonkin and Skirton, 2013; Calzone et al., 2010; Read and Ward, 2018). Some nurses have an awareness of the trajectory of genomic science including for example how whole genome sequencing might impact future health and care. Reading about current research such as the Generation Study, in which researchers are testing blood samples from neonates for genetic conditions, also helps nurses to think about what might be possible in the future and about their changing roles (Genomics England, 2024).

📖 Learning activity

- Read about the Genomics England Generation Study.
- Pick five of the conditions tested for, which you haven't previously read about, and search for further information about them including symptoms, how they are diagnosed and available treatments.

Overview of the Generation Study: https://www.generationstudy.co.uk/overview-of-the-study
    Conditions tested for in the Generation Study: https://www.generationstudy.co.uk/conditions-we-test-for/all-conditions

---

Core knowledge and skills

Genomics is a required competency for all registered nurses regardless of the area in which they work (Calzone et al., 2014). Knowledge related to 'genomics and the wider determinants of health' is a proficiency mandated by the UK Nursing and Midwifery Council (NMC, 2018, p.14). Most nurses now recognise the requirement for the modern workforce to have adequate genomic literacy, to understand the basics about genetics and disease and to be able to provide or facilitate the provision of necessary information, tests or care. This understanding includes DNA structure and function and the genetic contribution to disease or how genetic variation can increase the risk of some conditions within families and how this knowledge can be applied to practice to determine and manage these risks (Wright et al., 2019).

Unfamiliar terminology can be daunting but although they perceive their knowledge of genomics to be inadequate and may report feeling unprepared to deliver genomics related care, many nurses already perform genomics-related actions as part of their usual role (Wright et al., 2019). Nurses often ask people about their family history to inform other episodes of their care, facilitating discussion about inherited risk. Most have awareness of specific risks within a family health history in relation to the care provided, for example, contraception. Nurses will ask about heart attacks or strokes in first-degree relatives before supplying the combined oral contraceptive pill, owing to an increased risk of adverse drug reactions in women with certain risk factors such as a family history of cardiovascular conditions or events (Faculty of Sexual and Reproductive Health, 2023). However, nurses also need to develop the knowledge to act on such information beyond the current episode of care. This is because such information may also be significant in relation to future health.

An effective way of charting family health is to take and record a full family health history in order to organise information clearly so that it can be easily interpreted. When recording a family history, sometimes called a pedigree or family tree, nurses should have the ability to identify red flags which indicate the need to consider genomic testing (Bueser at al., 2022). Red flags are not diagnostic criteria but presenting factors which raise the suspicion of a possible underlying pathology. Identifying genomic red flags means recognising factors for individuals which may present a risk, for example any inherited cardiac conditions which could increase the risk of heart attack, or a family history of breast cancer. Patients who reveal a possible genetic pre-disposition for a specific condition may be referred to genomic specialists to initiate investigations that could lead to a diagnosis or early intervention and improve their health outcomes (Calzone et al., 2010).

Following discussion of the family history, communication skills are required to give clear, accurate information related to risk and to signpost patients to resources they can use to find more information which they can review at their own pace. Discussing and obtaining consent for a genomic referral, so that risk can be comprehensively assessed, tests requested and genetic counselling offered requires basic genomics skills and knowledge. In the first instance, for many people a discussion with their practice nurse or GP will provide some clarity on the next steps.

⚕ Skills focus – a step-by-step family health history:

- Start with the patient and their partner and children.
- Any miscarriages can be represented using triangles.
- Record their names and surnames (include the maiden names of females where possible to establish links to members of their birth families) and dates of birth (this will help when accessing their medical records if needed).
- Record sibling information for patient.
- Start to construct a larger family tree diagram, using circles to denote females and squares to denote males.

- Include the patient's mother and her siblings, her parents and their siblings. Then move on to the patient's father and his siblings, his parents and their siblings.
- Use horizontal lines to connect people by marriage and vertical lines to link parents and children.
- A strike through a person's circle or square symbol indicates that they are deceased, and it is useful to include their age of death.
- The ethnic ancestry of the persons included can also provide important information about genetic inheritance.
- Work backwards through the family to chart any significant health issues, one side at a time.
- Record the details of any conditions highlighted in the patient's own words (because some terms may be used to mean different things for example 'heart attack').
- It is useful to remember that problems which may seem unrelated may result from the same genetic variant manifesting in different ways. For example, Lynch syndrome, an inherited cancer pre-disposition syndrome, can cause different cancers.
- If indicated, ask about consanguinity or blood relationships between partners, which can increase the likelihood of passing on a genetic variant responsible for autosomal recessive conditions.
- Ask if there is anything else the patient thinks might be relevant.
- Ask about genetic red flags, including:
  - family members who developed health conditions at an unusually young age;
  - several members of the same biological family with same condition; and
  - unusual occurrences of conditions (such as breast cancer in males).

Adapted from Gen-Equip (2017).

Recognised symbols are used to indicate the biological sex of those included and horizontal and vertical lines are used to indicate whether people have the same parents or are related by marriage Figure 3.1). The symbols and nomenclature which denote sex have now been updated to include a diamond symbol for non-binary or gender diverse people and to indicate where clarity may be useful the gender which any person was assigned at birth (Bennett et al., 2022). It is important to record biological sex in addition to gender to ensure screening is offered when appropriate for sex-specific cancers, such as prostate cancer.

⚙ **Thinking point:**

- Why do you think it is necessary to include miscarriages on family health histories?
- In which situations do you think this information might be particularly significant?

Answering patient questions about genomics is becoming a more significant part of the nursing role in response to increased public awareness. Most people know that changes in some specific genes can cause breast cancer and that these genetic changes can be passed on within families. Celebrities often share their stories with the media and Angelina Jolie is a well-known example. Angelina Jolie inherited a BRCA gene variant from her mother

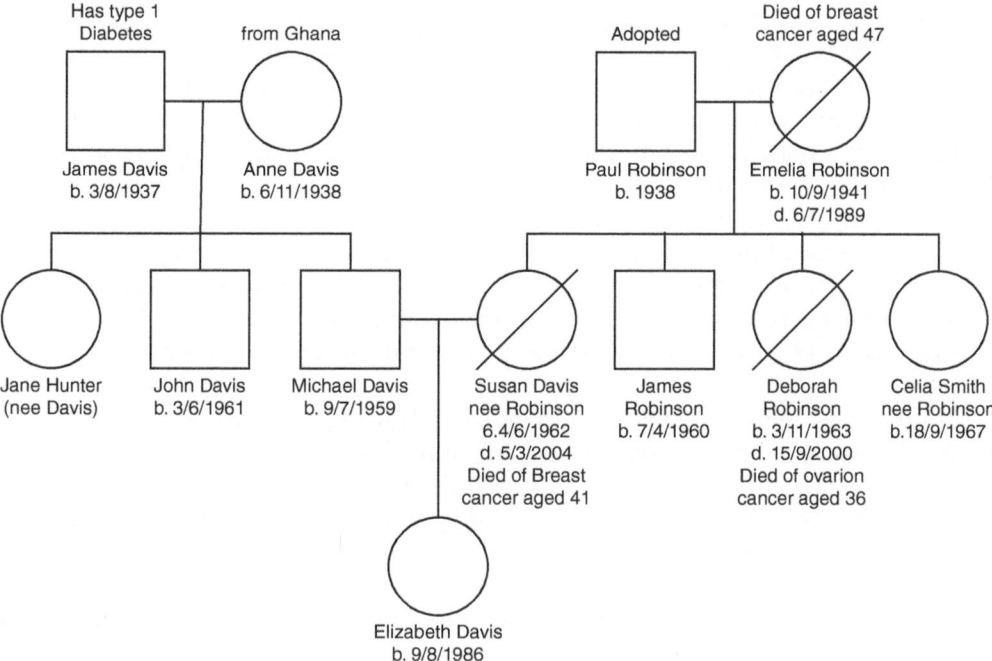

Figure 3.1 Example of a family health history.

and her decision to have prophylactic surgery to reduce her own risk was widely reported. Public interest in the story increased awareness regarding inherited risk and the rise in the number of women seeking genetic testing, which probably led to improved outcomes for many women, was referred to as the 'Angelina Jolie effect' (Orringer, 2018). Many people have friends or colleagues who have been affected by breast cancer and when attending for routine appointments, patients may use the opportunity to ask nurses in any setting about BRCA gene variations and about their own level of risk.

Questions from patients require all nurses to have a greater foundational knowledge of genetics than the general population. They must also have some general knowledge about which screening might be available and how to access tests or make onward referrals when appropriate. For example, a man can request a prostate specific antigen test from age 45 if there is a history of prostate cancer within his family. Nurses with basic genomic literacy can set patients on their journey towards early testing, diagnosis and treatment (Read and Ward, 2018). Breast screening is offered to women in the UK every 3 years between the ages 50 and 71 (NHS, 2021) but for some people, accessing screening sooner than usual might be recommended. Nurses can encourage early screening and regular routine self-examination when equipped with knowledge about increased risk. For example, BRCA gene testing is available to all UK citizens of Jewish ancestry over 18 as part of a targeted population screening approach to reduce certain cancers (NHS England, 2024). It is also necessary to inform first-degree male relatives of women with BRCA1 gene mutations about the gene's equal prevalence in men. This information is not widely known but nurses can prompt affected men to encourage their children to seek early screening (Read and Ward, 2018).

The impact of cultural, lifestyle and environmental factors on health is an integral part of genomics. Individual or combined factors such as smoking, poor diet or lack of exercise can affect a person's genes and alter their health. Understanding that complex conditions can occur as a result of inherited variation in one or more genes and the interaction of a person's genes with environmental harms helps nurses to promote health. Identifying specific vulnerabilities and delivering targeted health promotion can support people to protect themselves from epigenetic changes and lead to other health benefits. Patient education may take the form of methods and support for smoking cessation, increased exercise and better nutrition, or minimising exposure to UV rays from the sun. Routine discussion focused on lifestyle changes and promoting support services, for example at GP surgeries, also contributes to increased public awareness of common risks to health and protective measures. Posters and leaflets about genetic risks may also prompt questions about personalised medicine and the benefits of genomic testing.

Many nurses come into contact with individuals with genetic conditions at different points within their lifespan and in different clinical settings. As part of multidisciplinary care teams, nurses communicate regularly with other health care professionals and this communication is gradually expanding to include discussion about genomics related care (Wright et al., 2019). Discussion will be better informed by a good understanding of how some targeted treatments work and the required monitoring. Nurses in some settings may also have to integrate information from pharmacogenomic tests into patient treatment plans. As genomic medicine moves from specialist services to becoming part of mainstream care, or changes from a 'niche' to a 'necessity' discipline, nurses must build on their existing competence through recognising and addressing gaps in knowledge (North East and Yorkshire Genomic Medicine Service, 2023). This personal development encompasses the identification of genomic risk and testing to support a diagnosis but nurses in many settings are also required to care for patients and families already living with a genetic condition. Many routine episodes of care provide opportunities to identify the need for and to offer support through facilitating access to peer groups, social services, disability services and respite care.

Competency frameworks

Genomics knowledge including an awareness of the national testing infrastructure, the national strategy for developing genomic services and the direction of genomic advancement can assist nurses to understand the relevance of genomics to their role and to predict when nurses, nursing associates and student nurses are likely to be involved in patients' genomic journeys. As nursing practice changes and roles expand to incorporate genomics, education can help to extend knowledge and develop new skills such as recording a family health history and identifying genetic risk factors. The rapid pace of technological advancements in genomics has created challenges for nurse leaders regarding the prediction of competencies which nurses might need in this area and for nurse education in terms of integrating new content (Greco and Salveson, 2009). Nationally agreed competencies are necessary for safe and consistent practice within the diverse nursing workforce and competency frameworks provide a comprehensive list of skills in which nurses are required to become proficient (Calzone et al., 2014). The UK has a concise framework to guide registered nurses towards ensuring that they can provide optimal genomics care.

> ### ⚕ The 2023 Genomic Competency Framework for UK Nurses
>
> 1. Identify individuals who might benefit from genomic services and/or information as part of assessing needs and planning care.
> 2. Demonstrate effective communication in tailoring genomic information and services to the individual.
> 3. Advocate for the rights of all individuals to make informed decisions and act voluntarily.
> 4. Demonstrate a knowledge and understanding of genomics in human development, variation and health to underpin effective practice.
> 5. Apply knowledge, understanding and context of genomic testing and information to underpin care and support for individuals and families prior to, during and following decision-making.
> 6. Examine your own competency of practice on a regular basis.
> 7. Obtain and communicate reliable, current information about genomics, for self, patients, families and colleagues.
> 8. Provide ongoing nursing care and support to patients, carers, families and communities with genomic health care needs (NHS England, 2023).

Achieving competence – student nurses

Effective pre-registration genomics education can support nurses to maximise the benefits of genomics for patients and to ensure readiness for practice, education providers must ensure that:

- nursing programmes contain sufficient relevant genomics content;
- genomic concepts are linked to core nursing skills, for example that teaching about the inheritance patterns of common genetic conditions is linked to skills sessions on taking a family history; and
- there are strong links between taught theoretical content and student practice experiences (Calzone et al., 2010).

Genomics is included in the Nursing and Midwifery Council (NMC) 2018 standards of proficiency, but higher education institutions have the flexibility to interpret how students will be supported to achieve these standards, leading to variation in the skills and knowledge of newly qualified nurses. Genetics and genomics are often taught as part of bioscience modules, but a more integrated curricular thread can facilitate focus on how genomics affects all aspects of nursing; for example, genomics content can be easily included at relevant points in modules relating to pharmacology, ethics, oncology and communication skills. Curricular content to aligned to national competency frameworks can ensure adequate coverage of all necessary elements (Mathis, 2022).

Authentic interactions can help students to build the skills required to discuss genomics with real patients and linking theory to practice can help them to consider the impact of testing, diagnosis and living with genetic conditions on individuals and their families. Experiential learning also helps students to appreciate the individual nature of a person's genomics journey and how specific aspects will affect people differently within the context of their own belief systems. People will also have differing levels of understanding, and different personal situations, concerns and influencing factors, which affect how they cope with adversity. In addition to biosciences knowledge, nurse education must recognise the importance of skills for problem-solving and managing ethical questions in practice (Lea et al., 2011).

⚙ Supporting students

- Think of an episode of care within your clinical setting which could facilitate discussion with a student nurse about genetic and genomic contributions to health.
- If you are a student, consider how some of your practice learning proficiencies might be achieved in relation to any element of a patient's genomics journey.

Post-registration education

Nurses revalidate every 3 years to support continued competence in practice. This process can prompt them to consider accessing education and developing skills in response to any gaps impeding declarations of competence. Senior nurses must also feel sufficiently confident to support junior nurses and students to develop genomics knowledge and skills (Buaki-Sogo and Percival, 2022). Nurses should have an awareness that genomic information can lead to targeted early screening to help prevent disease and underpin decisions about precision treatment to improve outcomes (Calzone et al., 2014). However, it is reported that some nurses within today's nursing community are concerned that a historic lack of genomics-based content in their own curricula may put them at a disadvantage. Many nurses wish to maintain currency but feel that a lack of understanding may hinder them in incorporating genomic medicine into their practice (Bueser et al., 2022).

Both in the UK and internationally, numerous nurses would like to improve their competence and confidence in genomics-related care in line with developments in technology, to meet the needs of patients and their families. This means further understanding of the relevance of genomics to their role, but common barriers include a lack of post-registration education training opportunities which could help prepare the wider nursing community for the future. Registered nurses in many settings report that they would attend a genomics update or specific training if there was some available (Rahma et al., 2020). Targeted education and a focus on specialist career pathways are also seen as important for those wishing to work in genomics services (Calzone et al., 2018). Nurses are an important facet in the implementation of genetic testing within routine NHS care and as such they will require support to develop the proficiencies required to realise the benefits of genomics technologies for patients.

One specific example can be seen in relation to pharmacogenomics. Most nurses administer medications as part of their role and pharmacogenetic testing, which provides information about an individual's likely response to a medication, can increase patient safety in this area. Many nurses would like to develop the use of testing to benefit patients and feel that pharmacogenomics could be better integrated into health care systems if nurses had an increased understanding of testing utility and more confidence in requesting tests and managing results (Rahma et al., 2020). Nurses who have learned about pharmacogenomic testing in their pre- or post-registration training and who have the opportunity to incorporate information from such tests into care can better prevent and manage medication side effects to support patient adherence to medicines (Youssef et al., 2020). However, some nurses feel that inequalities in health and in health service provision in some areas can affect what is offered to their patients and delay their own professional development in terms of making relevant changes to their roles (Bueser et al., 2022).

The UK currently offers an educational framework consisting of a number of modules contributing to a Masters in Genomic Medicine which are delivered at a range of institutions (Health Education England, 2025A). The Genomics Education Programme education page (https://www.genomicseducation.hee.nhs.uk/education/?swoof=1&product_cat=taught-courses) lists a wide range of additional taught modules for a range of health professionals from Fundamentals in Human Genetics and Genomics, Genomics and Counselling Skills to Genomics of Common Neurological Disorders.

Other challenges for nurses wishing to access education, however, include overstretched services and staff shortages, which mean that managers feel that they cannot agree to time away from clinical roles for study. Despite system pressures, clear strategies to develop the nursing workforce including a commitment from organisational managers to provide a budget and time out for training would provide the means to address knowledge deficits.

📖 Learning activity

- Reflect upon your own core nursing skills and write down the skills you think you already have which would help you to support patients on their genomics journeys.
- Next, write down the skills you think it is important to develop in this area as services evolve.

(This learning activity is designed to support achievement of NHS England (2023) genomic nursing competency 6.)

Integrating genomics into practice

Effective resources can enable nurse competency in genomics through the development of knowledge and skills in genomics care (Calzone et al., 2014). NHS England has provided the Genomics Education Programme (GEP) which includes free resources for nurses practising at all levels. The GEP resource includes a section titled 'GeNotes' which is home to the useful 'Knowledge Hub'. The Knowledge Hub (https://www.genomicseducation.hee.nhs.uk/genotes/knowledge-hub/) is an encyclopaedia of resources designed to support understanding of genomics in health care. This multi-professional resource incorporates accessible bitesize education to suit busy professionals. Topics covered include for example information about the structure and function of DNA, information relating to specific conditions and therapies, and information about new technologies for example in relation to whole genome sequencing.

Knowledge focus – inheritance patterns

Autosomal recessive conditions

Mathilde has 2 daughters and Emilie, the eldest of the two, has a child with sickle cell disease. Mathilde's youngest daughter, Sophie, is pregnant and Mathilde asks her practice nurse, Bobbi about the risk of Sophie's child also being born with sickle cell disease.

Bobbi knows that sickle cell disease is inherited in an autosomal recessive pattern. The child will only be at risk if there is a likelihood that both parents are carriers of a variation in the HBB gene. She needs to establish the blood relationships to the child of people in the family who either have Sickle cell disease or have a child with the condition. To do this she constructs a family tree.

Bobbi then feels equipped to share accurate information about the baby's risk with Mathilde. (Adapted from Read and Ward, 2018.)

Other common conditions inherited in an autosomal recessive pattern include:

- sickle cell anaemia
- cystic fibrosis
- Tay–Sachs disease
- spinal muscular atrophy.

Autosomal dominant conditions

Later that week, Bobbi sees Harrison, who is 5 and has come in for a regular developmental check. Harrison has Marfan syndrome. Bobbi knows that Harrison's father, Richard, doesn't have the condition but that Harrison has inherited Marfan syndrome because his mother Becky does. Although it can occur spontaneously, Marfan syndrome is usually inherited in an autosomal dominant pattern and inheriting the faulty FBN1 gene from only one parent has resulted in Harrison being born with this condition.

Richard and Becky's other child, George, aged 9, does not have the condition, which means that he inherited Becky's normal copy of the gene without the mutation that causes Marfan syndrome.

Other common conditions inherited in an autosomal dominant pattern include:

- Huntington's disease
- Marfan syndrome
- polycystic kidney disease
- neurofibromatosis.

X-linked conditions

Boys inherit an X-chromosome from their biological mother and a Y-chromosome from their father, which determines their biological sex. One of Bobbi's other regular patients is Daniel, aged 12, who has Duchenne muscular dystrophy. This disease is caused by a faulty gene in the X-chromosome, which can be passed on from mother to child. Boys usually develop the disease when they inherit the faulty gene because they do not have a second X-chromosome to make up for lost function whereas girls may inherit the faulty gene but have only mild symptoms. Daniel has routine appointments with Bobbi to review his pain medication review and to check the integrity of his skin as he has difficulty with mobility and usually uses a wheelchair.

X-Linked conditions can be recessive or dominant and some others include:

■ haemophilia
■ red–green colour blindness
■ fragile X syndrome
■ Rett syndrome.

Familial hypercholesterolaemia

In UK and international health services, the incidence of drug treatment being led by the results of genomic tests is increasing and prescribing guided by genetic information is improving outcomes (Lea et al., 2011). For this reason, nurses need to develop an awareness of how test results can directly affect treatment planning. Familial hyper-cholesterolaemia is an example of a condition that illustrates this well.

If a person has a cardiac event before they are 50, they should be offered a test for a condition called familial hypercholesterolaemia (FH). Familial hypercholesterolae-mia occurs owing to a hereditary genetic variation causing interruption to the body's normal process for metabolising low-density lipoprotein (LDL) cholesterol. Familial hypercholesterolaemia is an autosomal dominant disorder which leads to hyperlipi-daemia (elevated blood lipid levels). Clinical management of FH is usually provided through specialist lipid clinics to manage cholesterol levels by providing treatment which replaces the function lost through genetic variation. Treatment is usually sta-tin therapy alongside the clinical management of high blood pressure. Drugs can be used in combination with diet and lifestyle changes to improve prognosis and decrease health risks caused by atheroma (fatty deposits in the arteries).

If a person is diagnosed with a condition that has an autosomal dominant inherit-ance pattern, approximately half of their first-degree relatives will also have it and should be offered testing (Ned and Sijbrands, 2011). Familial hypercholesterolaemia has an estimated prevalence of 1 in 200–500 in European populations but is vastly underdiagnosed and when left untreated can result in premature coronary artery disease and increase the risk of myocardial infarction. This means that care settings must improve the mechanism through which people with FH are currently identified (Humphries et al., 2018). Reviewing all patients in GP practices who have ever had a total cholesterol of over 9 mmol/l to exclude secondary causes and then offering a refer-ral to lipid clinic for assessment may help (Heart UK, 2025).

Children can be diagnosed with FH and should be tested where indicated. If diag-nosed, family lipid clinics can facilitate access to care and improve outcomes. The Child–Parent Screening Service was a pilot service development programme which ran between 2022 and 2024. The programme identified children and parents with FH through heel prick tests performed at routine 1 year immunisation visits (Health Innovation North East and North Cumbria, 2024). Genetic information can also be obtained using a mouth swab, and application of the Simon Broome diagnostic criteria can enable health care practitioners to determine whether a patient has likely or definite FH. This tool contains questions about family history of cardiovascular events in combination with cholesterol levels and information from testing for genetic variants. The Simon Broome criteria also take into account cholesterol deposits around the tendons (xanthomas, often appearing on the joints). These deposits can also appear around the eyes (xanthelasmas) (MD CALC, 2024).

Information from routine consultations in the primary care setting which is identified as a 'red flag' or potential indicator and appropriately acted upon can lead to a genomic test, potential early diagnosis and treatment of a genetic condition. Detection of FH can reduce cardiovascular risks associated with high cholesterol levels. High LDL cholesterol levels have also been shown to increase the risk of dementia in later life (Livingston et al., 2024).

⚑ Red flags for genetic conditions

- A strong family history of a condition (especially cancers or cardiac or cardiovascular conditions).
- A patient who is unusually young to have specific symptoms or the condition you suspect.
- A patient in whom the symptoms of a condition are unusually severe.
- An absence of environmental factors usually associated with a condition.
- Any sudden or early deaths reported within a patient's family.
- An infant or child with a combination of unusual symptoms.
- A child with similar health problems to somebody else in their family.

Adapted from Primary Care Genetics (2017).

In 2023, the Genomics Education Programme introduced the Clinical Pathway Initiative (CPI). This resource outlines clinical pathways, focusing on the key competencies required of health professionals at each stage of a patient's genomics journey. The CPIs support a unified and consistent approach to the integration of genomics across different clinical specialties within UK health care systems and can be useful in the development of nurse led genomic services. Specialist nurses were instrumental in developing these adaptable guidelines and the FH pathway summarises key steps to guide effective practice. The CPIs support nurses in specified settings to identify their learning needs, for example assessment of genetic risk and to consider the associated resources through which they can address knowledge deficits. Specialist nursing roles within genomics services are explored further in Chapter 4.

📖 Learning activity

- Explore the Genomics Education Programme CPI for Familial Hypercholesterolemia (https://www.genomicseducation.hee.nhs.uk/the-clinical-pathway-initiative/cpi-familial-hypercholesterolaemia/).

■ Identify which of the listed competencies you have or would like to develop to enhance your role.

■ List ways in which you could develop the skills that you identified and any support you could ask for from your employer.

🔍 Case study – familial hypercholesterolaemia

On Friday evening, Phil, aged 55, calls his GP out of hours service. He is worried because he has experienced sporadic mild chest pain for two days and a brief episode of arm weakness this afternoon which has now resolved. He is referred to the Urgent Care Centre where he is assessed to determine whether he might have had a heart attack or a stroke. Phil starts to feel better and after a number of cardiac, cardiovascular and neurological investigations which did not reveal anything of concern, he is discharged home.

After a few days, Phil receives a telephone call from the Urgent Care Centre. The person he speaks to tells him that the blood tests he had on Friday showed his LDL cholesterol to be well above the normal range (below 5 mmol/L) at 7 mmol/L.

Phil makes an appointment to see the practice nurse, Debbie, at his GP surgery and she prescribes him atorvastatin which reduces the synthesis of cholesterol in the liver. At the appointment, Debbie asks Phil whether there is any history of high cholesterol levels or cardiac conditions within his family. Phil reports that his dad died from a heart attack aged 57 and tells Debbie that he is worried that he might have a heart condition, even though nothing significant was identified at the Urgent Care Centre.

Debbie explains her suspicions regarding FH with Phil and gives him some information about the condition. They discuss the option to test for FH and the implications of a positive result for Phil and his family. Phil consents to a referral for genetic counselling at the local hospital's FH clinic.

At the clinic, the FH Nurse uses the Simon Broome criteria to assess Phil, which indicates 'possible' FH which would become 'definite' if supported by genetic information. He confirms Phil's eligibility for the test against the criteria listed in the National Genomic Test Directory and obtains informed consent from Phil to send a blood sample for testing.

The test comes back positive for a genetic variant which can cause FH. The management of Phil's treatment is taken over by the FH clinic under the care of the specialist nurse. Phil has 2 daughters who are offered appointments at the clinic.

Phil sends the practice nurse Debbie a Thank You card because her successful identification of his genomic risk led to treatment to reduce his risk and also helped to reduce his anxiety.

Health promotion

Prevention of harm is inherent within genomic health care and nurses are well positioned to deliver health promotion education. Frequent contact with patients and the unique insights offered by patients to nurses can help to capitalise on nursing strengths in this area of practice (Calzone et al., 2010). A good understanding of how environmental factors affect the genome can inform nursing care and nurses can motivate patients to make positive changes by identifying risk and discussing key research evidence in targeted genomics-based health promotion (Tonkin and Skirton, 2013). For example, the risk of age-related macular degeneration is increased by genetic factors in combination with lifestyle factors like smoking, diet and obesity and help to reduce environmental contributors and introduce protective factors, such as exercise, healthy diet and sleep hygiene can be beneficial.

🩺 Skills focus – smoking cessation

Referring patients to NHS services to support them to stop smoking greatly increases their chance of success:

- Services are run by expert advisors who can provide clear information and evidence-based support for the first few months.
- Patients can access one-to-one appointments with advisors and sessions are available by phone or video call for those who cannot attend a clinic.
- Advisors can help patients to design a plan to quit that best suits them.
- They can also provide nicotine replacement therapies and the use of other tools.
- Support is also provided for when people relapse to help them to sustain the motivation to give up smoking (NHS, 2022).

In addition to the impact of a person's lifestyle on their genes, the genes they are born with can also affect the relationship between a person's diet and their health. Recognising causal connections between diet, gene expression and health outcomes means that nurses can give targeted information about nutrition when required. Chemicals in some processed foods and nutritional deficiencies can cause changes to a person's genome and increase their susceptibility to disease. Obesity also increases the risk of associated conditions such as diabetes, joint problems, cardiovascular conditions and low mood (Prasad et al., 2011).

Epigenetic changes

Epigenetics concerns the parts of the genome that aren't DNA. Methylation or the addition of methyl group chemicals (sometimes called chemical markers) to DNA does not modify the DNA sequence itself but can affect gene expression – whether certain genes are switched on or off. The body uses methyl groups from food to ensure that genes which are not needed at different stages of the lifespan are switched off by preventing the transcription of DNA and the formation of new proteins. This is a key reason why health promotion concerning adequate nutrition is important.

Methyl groups can also come from toxic substances like smoking or environmental chemicals, and this can disrupt normal methylation patterns. When some genes are switched off inappropriately, for example genes which function to prevent diseases like cancer from developing, diseases can develop more freely. Some genes inhibit abnormal cell growth and without these genes abnormal cells can grow to form tumours. Lynch syndrome is an inherited pre-cancer syndrome which increases the risk of developing some cancers within families. If a person with Lynch syndrome introduces lifestyle factors such as smoking, they increase their vulnerability to these cancers. Additional information about Lynch syndrome and the nursing role can be found in Chapter 4.

Child development

There are multiple genes that regulate neurodevelopment and methylation to these genes can affect the growth and development of infants and children. Excessive alcohol use in pregnancy can cause changes to foetal DNA, causing babies to be born with foetal alcohol syndrome and associated developmental delay. If methylation occurs in childhood some of the genes that regulate neurodevelopment can be switched off and affect a child's functioning and the rate at which they reach their developmental milestones (Harvard University Center on the Developing Child, 2019).

Traumatic early life experiences including instability at home or 'toxic stressors' such as neglect or abuse can also affect the epigenome or the arrangement of chemical markers which affect gene expression and change how a child develops by altering their normal physiological responses to stress (Magalhães-Barbosa et al., 2022). Such changes can affect a child's behaviours and achievement and understanding the potential impact of early life experiences on the epigenome (epigenomics) and the impact of parental care on infant health and development can help child nurses to support parents more effectively. Research has shown that structured nursing interventions, particularly in areas of socio-economic deprivation, can improve pre-natal health, parenting skills and child health and well-being. Intervention could take the form of visiting the home and providing family-centred care. It is also important to identify pre- or post-natal depression as quickly as possible (Gonzalez et al., 2018).

Skills focus – When a parent appears to be or discloses that they are struggling

- Listen with empathy and without judgement.
- Show compassion and reassure parents that most parents experience challenges.
- Give education and practical advice – this could be related to fostering good sleep patterns, or coping mechanisms if they have a new baby and are struggling to form a routine.
- Talk about their own support networks such as parents and friends, or maybe other parents if they have an older child.
- Give accessible written information to take away.
- Let them know how they can contact you again if they feel overwhelmed and book a follow-up appointment in the near future.
- Refer them to other useful support services, this might be a social needs assessment from the local council if their child is disabled or a peer support group.

It is important for nurses to recognise their safeguarding responsibilities and to consider any risk of harm to a child. Any nurse should contact their local safeguarding team to discuss concerns if they have them. It is the duty of all staff working in health care to:

- identify problems quickly;
- provide help and support to meet the needs of children as soon as any problems are identified;
- protect children from maltreatment;
- prevent impairment of child mental and physical health and development.

(Adapted from HM Government, 2023.)

Equality, diversity and inclusion

Newer understanding of genetic pre-disposition to disease contributes not only to effective screening, early diagnosis and early and effective treatment for individuals but also to disease management in the general population (Matthews-Juarez and Juarez, 2011). To practise within modern health care services, nurses require literacy in genomics and the support to foster inclusive practice. Nursing tools for inclusive practice include cultural competence and the consideration of groups of diverse origin within communities who might benefit from genomics related information or care. This is an important point because at present, not all ethnic populations in the UK are benefitting equally from developments in genomic medicine (Brigden and Krishnan, 2023).

Learning about different cultures and recognising increased genetic vulnerability in some ethnic populations can help nurses to mitigate risk. Nurses should also acquire knowledge relating to genetic conditions more prevalent within specific ethnicities including sickle cell disease in those with African genetic heritage – more detail on sickle cell disease can be found in Chapter 4. In some community groups there is also an elevated risk of developing or dying from some common conditions such as heart disease, and nurses who work in UK communities with large South Asian populations should be aware of the increased risk of coronary heart disease. Both men and women with Indian, Pakistani, Bangladeshi and Sri Lankan heritage can develop heart disease at an earlier age and are more likely to be hospitalised, and their mortality risk is greater than that of the general population (Pursnani and Merchant, 2020).

All nurses require knowledge of social and cultural determinants of health. Consanguinity, or the practice of marrying first cousins, is a custom which creates an increased probability of transmitting genetic conditions within families (Greco and Salveson, 2009). Consanguinity leads to an increased risk of congenital malformations and autosomal recessive metabolic conditions, caused by alterations to enzymes involved in metabolic pathways. This practice can also increase susceptibility to complex disorders in later life with factors such as obesity, diabetes, cardiovascular conditions and some cancers contributing to this risk (Oniya et al., 2019). It is, however, important not to make assumptions or to generalise and the practice of consanguinity does not cause problems if neither parent has or is a carrier of a genetic condition or syndrome. Appreciating how one's own beliefs, values and biases can affect any care delivered is an essential part of the nursing role.

The knowledge and sensitivity of individual nurses can help many individuals, but culturally competent care systems make the biggest difference in reducing health disparities and the impact of these disparities on disadvantaged groups. Effective regional services can influence factors such as infant mortality rates, average time to diagnosis and the prevalence and severity of long-term conditions. Culturally competent health services understand ethnic populations and cultural norms, which may contribute to behaviours around health, and recognise how social disadvantages affect how and when different minority groups will access care (Matthews-Juarez and Juarez, 2011). Care should be designed and implemented with sensitivity to practical needs based on cultural influences and values within local communities in order to provide equity of care, for example facilitating attendance in groups and offering a choice of health care practitioner based on gender. Such planning requires detailed knowledge about the local community and population groups. Culturally competent care is explored further in Chapter 6, which considers ethical issues including genomic health inequality.

Black people, those from ethnic minority groups and people from marginalised groups such as those from LGBTQI communities may not often be given the opportunity or may often decline to participate in health research (Bueser et al., 2022, Matthews-Juarez and Juarez, 2011). It is a responsibility of the nursing community to facilitate inclusion and participation in genomic research to increase available data and advances in the field. There is currently a disproportionate amount of data available from people of European ancestry and better representation from diverse participants will improve the generalis-ability of study findings to benefit more patient groups, especially in terms of responses to medications, which can vary between different ethnicities (Bueser et al., 2022). A lack of data from non-European populations about responses to some medicines can lead to the prescription of sub-therapeutic doses or supra-therapeutic doses, which increase the risk of medication side effects (Brigden and Krishnan, 2023). Further information about pharmacogenomics in relation to different populations can be found in Chapter 7.

Complex diseases
Genomics is no longer confined to clinical genetics services and has begun to influence many other aspects of care (Wright et al., 2019). Genomic health care increasingly involves predicting and mitigating risk factors for common diseases, especially those with multiple contributing lifestyle and genetic factors. Such conditions include schizo-phrenia, diabetes, heart disease, Parkinson's disease, hypertension, coronary artery disease and some common cancers.

Nurses must learn how to identify polygenic risk or the risk of patients developing one or more conditions caused by the combination of variations in multiple genes, often strongly influenced by behavioural and environmental factors. The long-term response to cigarette smoking, for example, can be different in many individuals, partly down to smoking behaviours but also owing to individual differences in the inflammatory response to cigarette smoke. Smoking may or may not lead to chronic obstructive pulmonary disease (COPD) based on a person's genetic make-up. There are a number of genes in which variation and changes can increase susceptibility to developing COPD or to the severity of symptoms among different people, different families and different races (Liu et al., 2022).

With some multifactorial disorders it may be possible to predict an individual's risk of developing certain symptoms and conditions and polygenic risk scores are being developed to help predict an individual's risk of developing a complex disease. Further information about polygenic risk scores can be found in Chapter 5. An understanding of how genomic factors contribute to increased susceptibility to certain diseases can help support nurses in any area of care to deliver effective health promotion. Information about lifestyle changes can make a positive difference and for some, discussion related to screening or the initiation of treatment may be appropriate. Many skilled interventions are required to plan care for those with a variety of needs relating to complex conditions and nurses work in collabora-tion with multidisciplinary teams to meet these needs.

MODY
Maturity onset diabetes of the young (MODY) is a form of diabetes which often presents in adolescence or early adulthood and is usually diagnosed before the age of 25. This con-dition is caused by the inheritance of a pathogenic mutation in one of a number of possible

genes and is inherited in an autosomal dominant pattern. It is a rare form of diabetes, different from both type 1 and type 2 diabetes, and this condition runs strongly in families. Diabetic ketoacidosis is not usually a feature of MODY. If a parent has a MODY-causing gene mutation, any child they have has a 50% chance of inheriting it from them.

MODY is frequently misdiagnosed which can lead to incorrect treatment, but early and accurate diagnosis can vastly improve care and patient experience (Shepherd et al., 2014). Unlike type 1 diabetes which is an autoimmune (rather than genetic) condition which inhibits insulin production in the pancreas, some people who have MODY still produce insulin, meaning that treatment with insulin is not indicated and may cause harm. For example, HNF1α MODY (MODY caused by a mutation on the HNF1α gene) is responsive to low dose sulfonylureas, such as gliclazide or glimepiride, which stimulate the pancreas to produce insulin (Diabetes Genes, 2025). This helps to avoid hypoglycaemic episodes, common in type 1 diabetes, and also to avoid the need for frequent blood glucose tests. Nurses prepared with this knowledge can be vigilant for cases of type 1 or 2 diabetes with any atypical features and initiate testing for MODY.

Some gestational diabetes can also be caused by MODY gene mutations and most neonatal diabetes is MODY (Kleinberger and Pollin, 2015). The right test followed by timely and correct interpretation can lead to better relative outcomes for these patients. The Genetic Diabetes Nurse project, established in 2002, has been instrumental in increasing awareness about MODY for health care professionals across the UK; referral rates for tests have increased and families have been receiving the support they need as result of effective diagnosis and treatment (Shepherd et al., 2014).

🔍 Case study

Lena, aged 23, is fit and active and her body mass index is within the normal range. Her father was diagnosed with type 2 diabetes aged 54.

Lena presents at her GP surgery with recurrent vaginal candidiasis (thrush) and polyuria. She has not experienced any weight gain or weight loss. The practice nurse notes glycosuria on urinalysis and proceeds to test Lena's blood glucose levels, which are raised.

Some blood samples are sent to the lab and while she has an unexpectedly low haemoglobin A1C (HbA1c) level, Lena is told that she has diabetes. She is prescribed insulin and taught how to monitor her blood glucose levels. She also receives advice about maintaining a healthy lifestyle.

Over the next few months, the insulin makes no difference to Lena's high blood glucose levels. She also experiences frequent hypoglycaemic episodes throughout which she is dizzy and shaky and has palpitations. Lena becomes increasingly anxious and makes an appointment to have the dose of her medication reviewed.

The nurse Lena sees has immediate suspicions regarding MODY owing to Lena's unusual story. She thinks that the insulin she has been given has been supressing Lena's natural insulin and causing her hypos. They discuss the condition and what it might mean for Lena if she was diagnosed with it, and Lena consents to a referral to specialist services for a MODY test.

A few weeks later, Lena receives a positive diagnosis from a specialist nurse and her insulin is discontinued. This nurse discusses the implications of the genetic result and sharing information with her wider family. Lena is prescribed instead treatment targeted to the individual characteristics of her condition.

Since she has some endogenous insulin production, Lena's MODY is responsive to a low-dose sulfonylurea (gliclazide). Her glycaemic control improves, and she has no further hypos.

The nurse at Lena's GP surgery thinks about integrating consideration of MODY testing into care pathways for all suspected diabetes criteria. She creates a step in the surgery's computerised template to prompt practitioners to consider MODY when investigations for diabetes are initiated if appropriate, based on patient age, body mass index and HbA1c levels.

(Based on information from Colclough and Patel, 2022.)

Developing new clinical pathways

To optimise the benefit of new genomics technologies, accessing these technologies must become a routine part of care pathways in a greater number of services. Nurses can act as agents of change to support the integration of genomics effectively into existing services through the design and introduction of new steps within existing processes to prompt the consideration and discussion of genetic or genomic risk, genomics testing and referral to other services (Calzone et al., 2018).

As the focus on personalised and precision medicine increases, it is essential for the nursing profession to be involved in expanding and improving existing care provision. Nurses are skilled in the identification of patient needs and can advocate for patients so that services evolve to meet these needs. Nurses who recognise those who would benefit from genomics information or care can include these groups in service design, for example, women attending the emergency department and admitted to gynaecology wards following a miscarriage. The National Genomic Test Directory test R318 (NHS England, 2025, p.105) includes recurrent miscarriage (defined as three or more miscarriages) in the criteria for a genomic test if the products of conception are available for testing. Genetic factors are main cause of early miscarriage and nurses in gynaecology settings who are aware of this can ask about any previous miscarriages and retain any products of conception which can be tested for aneuploidy (an abnormal number of chromosomes) (Jia et al., 2015). Determining a possible reason for multiple miscarriages can help some women to cope with loss and may inform a woman or couple's family planning decisions.

Another example of where testing can be introduced into care pathways for specific patients relates to critical care nursing. When long QT syndrome is discovered in critical care settings, testing to determine a genetic cause should be considered and discussed with patients where possible and their families if a test is deemed appropriate. When other causes (such as medication side effects) can be ruled out, integrating a genomic test (test R127) into care pathways can provide vital information about the causes of disease (NHS England, 2025, p17). If a condition is genetic, even if it is identified following the unexpected death of the patient, there will be implications for the patient's family. In such cases, skilled advocacy may be required to meet health needs sensitively and effectively (Howington et al., 2011).

Including genomics within existing services may mean designing and implementing a pathway which includes the points at which testing might be discussed and any essential or optional actions based on the outcome of discussion. Process maps or flow charts can help to visualise the stages of each care pathway and to streamline patient journeys. As services change, nurses must be involved in writing local clinical protocols and guidelines when integrating genomics into services to ensure that any new processes work effectively for patients (Kirk et al., 2011). Process maps can also help to determine staff roles and overall time frames based on the estimated time between steps.

Accessing, interpreting and applying the law, for example in relation to organisational requirements for data privacy, is an essential part of designing processes and guidance from existing local policies can be useful. New processes should also be underpinned by appropriate research evidence to inform the development of each stage (Kirk et al., 2011). As with any service improvement, new genomics systems and processes must also be evaluated to identify areas for further improvement. When thinking about how any new elements of a service will run it is necessary to ensure that there are options for accessing them which support inclusivity for all patient groups. Patients can be asked for their feedback on this and other areas to help to evaluate services.

The specialist genomics workforce has been instrumental in developing the UK CPI to unify approaches to genomics related care in clinical settings within different organisations (Health Education England, 2025B). Changes to health services must be supported by strategic planning with regard to the role of the nurse, and nurse education and service level policies and training on how to use them should be considered when introducing new responsibilities into a nursing job description (Lopes-Júnior et al., 2022). Regional genomic medicine service alliances support health care teams across the UK by providing education and training, and their contact details can be found easily online (Buaki-Sogo and Percival, 2022). It is important for managers to identify any new skills which will be required by the nurses working within services and to consider how they will support their development. An example of this might include training on when and how to refer patients to other professionals. Case-based training or simulation might be useful to explore different situations and develop problem-solving skills including the ability to identify, address and manage ethical questions. Some examples of ethical issues associated with genomics are explored further in Chapter 6. Simulated patient interactions also help to practice giving accurate information.

Summary
The effective integration of genomic medicine depends upon nurses in all settings becoming familiar with key genomics concepts and terminology. This means addressing any gaps in understanding and being clear about how genomics is relevant to nursing practice. It also means accessing self-development opportunities to obtain new knowledge and skills to enhance practice, including the ability to discuss genetic and genomic risk and next steps with confidence. Nurses must keep up to date with current genomics research and consider how new developments might shape services to prepare for the future.

Genomics resources for nurses
The following is a list of free resources which can support nurses to develop knowledge and skills in genomics care:

■ The US National Human Genome Research Institute provides on online repository of peer-reviewed educational materials for health care professionals: https://www.genome.gov/GenomeEd/resources

- The One in Six Billion podcasts provide interesting and valuable insight into patient experiences of genetic forms of diabetes: https://1in6b.com/
- 'Let's Talk About Genomic Testing' is a series of six films that has been developed to cover the key points health care professionals need to consider when discussing genomic testing with patients and their families: https://www.genomicseducation. hee.nhs.uk/news/lets-talk-about-genomic-testing/
- The international society of nurses in genetics has a repository of useful resources for the nursing community: https://www.isong.org/
- This 'core principles' resource within the Genomics Education Programme links nursing and midwifery proficiencies to key learning resources: https://www.genomics education.hee.nhs.uk/wp-content/uploads/2023/09/Core-principles-document_ v4.pdf
- For practice assessors and other nurses supporting students, Health Education England (2021) provides examples of genomics care which can be linked to NMC (2018) proficiencies: https://www.genomicseducation.hee.nhs.uk/wp-content/uploads/ 2021/04/NMC-standards-genomics_14-04-21.pdf

Resources for patients
- An educational booklet for people with Familia Hypercholesterolaemia can be found at Heart UK: https://www.heartuk.org.uk/downloads/health-professionals/ publications/familial-hypercholesterolaemia.pdf

References

Bennett, R.L., French, K.S., Resta, R.G. and Austin, J., 2022. Practice resource-focused revision: standardized pedigree nomenclature update centered on sex and gender inclusivity: a practice resource of the National Society of genetic counselors. *Journal of Genetic Counseling*, 31(6), pp.1238–1248.

Brigden, Tanya and Krishnan, Bhavya, 2023. How do we close the diversity gap in genomics? https://www.phgfoundation.org/blog/how-do-we-close-the-diversity-gap-in-genomics/ (accessed 21 January, 2025).

Buaki-Sogo, M. and Percival, N., 2022. Genomic medicine: the role of the nursing workforce. *Nursing Times*, 118, pp.1–3.

Bueser, T., Skinner, A., Bolton Saghdaoui, L. and Moorley, C., 2022. Genomic research: the landscape for nursing. *Journal of Advanced Nursing*, 78(9), e99–e100.

Calzone, K.A., Cashion, A., Feetham, S., Jenkins, J., Prows, C.A., Williams, J.K. and Wung, S.F., 2010. Nurses transforming health care using genetics and genomics. *Nursing Outlook*, 58(1), pp.26–35.

Calzone, K.A., Jenkins, J., Culp, S., Caskey, S. and Badzek, L., 2014. Introducing a new competency into nursing practice. *Journal of Nursing Regulation*, 5(1), p.40.

Calzone, K.A., Kirk, M., Tonkin, E., Badzek, L., Benjamin, C. and Middleton, A. The global landscape of nursing and genomics. *Journal of nursing scholarship*. 2018 May;50(3):249–56.

Campion, M., Goldgar, C., Hopkin, R.J., Prows, C.A. and Dasgupta, S., 2019. Genomic education for the next generation of health-care providers. *Genetics in Medicine*, 21(11), pp.2422–2430.

Colclough, K. and Patel, K., 2022. How do I diagnose maturity onset diabetes of the young in my patients? *Clinical Endocrinology*, 97(4), pp.436–447.

Diabetes Genes, 2025. Hepatic Nuclear Factor 1 Alpha (HNF1A). https://www.diabetesgenes. org/what-is-mody/hepatic-nuclear-factor-1-alpha-hnf1a/ (accessed 30 January 2025).

Faculty of Sexual and Reproductive Health, 2023. Combined oral contraception. https://www.fsrh.org/Common/Uploaded%20files/documents/fsrh-guideline-combined-hormonal-contraception-october-2023.pdf (accessed 24 January 2025).

Gen-Equip, 2017. Taking an appropriate family history to detect possible genetic conditions. https://www.primarycaregenetics.org/?page_id=685&lang=en (accessed 29 May 2025).

Genomics England, 2024. Generation study. https://www.generationstudy.co.uk/overview-of-the-study (accessed 6 February 2025).

Gonzalez, A., Catherine, N., Boyle, M., Jack, S.M., Atkinson, L., Kobor, M., Sheehan, D., Tonmyr, L., Waddell, C. and MacMillan, H.L., 2018. Healthy Foundations Study: a randomised controlled trial to evaluate biological embedding of early-life experiences. *BMJ Open*, 8(1), p.e018915.

Greco, K.E. and Salveson, C., 2009. Identifying genetics and genomics nursing competencies common among published recommendations. *Journal of Nursing Education*, 48(10), pp.557–565.

Harvard University Center on the Developing Child, 2019. Epigenetics and child development: how children's experiences affect their genes. https://developingchild.harvard.edu/resources/what-is-epigenetics-and-how-does-it-relate-to-child-development/ (accessed 30 January 2025).

Health Education England, 2021. NMC proficiencies: relevance to genomic practice. https://www.genomicseducation.hee.nhs.uk/wp-content/uploads/2021/04/NMC-standards-genomics_14-04-21.pdf

Health Education England, 2025A. Genomics education programme. https://www.genomicseducation.hee.nhs.uk/about-us/masters-in-genomic-medicine/ (accessed 24 January, 2025).

Health Education England (2025B) Clinical Pathways Initiative. https://www.genomicseducation.hee.nhs.uk/the-clinical-pathway-initiative/ (accessed 29 May 2025).

Health Innovation North East and North Cumbria, 2024. Child-parent screening. https://healthinnovationnenc.org.uk/what-we-do/improving-population-health/cardiovascular-disease-prevention/familial-hypercholesterolaemia-fh/child-parent-screening/ (accessed 29 January 2025).

Heart UK, 2025. Familial hypercholesterolaemia. https://www.heartuk.org.uk/educational-content/fh-educational-materials (accessed 29 January 2025).

HM Government, 2023. Working together to safeguard children. https://assets.publishing.service.gov.uk/media/669e7501ab418ab055592a7b/Working_together_to_safeguard_children_2023.pdf (accessed 30 January 2025).

Howington, L., Riddlesperger, K. and Cheek, D.J., 2011. Essential nursing competencies for genetics and genomics: implications for critical care. *Critical Care Nurse*, 31(5), pp.e1–e7.

Humphries, S.E., Cooper, J.A., Seed, M., Capps, N., Durrington, P.N., Jones, B., McDowell, I.F.W., Soran, H., Neil, H.A.W. and Simon Broome Familial Hyperlipidaemia Register Group, 2018. Coronary heart disease mortality in treated familial hypercholesterolaemia: update of the UK Simon Broome FH register. *Atherosclerosis*, 274, pp.41–46.

Jia, C.-W., Wang, L., Lan, Y.-L., Song, R., Zhou, L.-Y., Yu, L., Yang, Y., Liang, Y., Li, Y., Ma, Y.-M. and Wang, S.-Y., 2015. Aneuploidy in early miscarriage and its related factors. *Chinese Medical Journal*, 128(20), pp.2772–2776.

Kirk, M., Campalani, S., Doris, F., Heron, J., Mannion, G., Metcalfe, A., Patch, C., Permalloo, N., Shepherd, M. and Calzone, K., 2011. Genetics/genomics in nursing and midwifery: Task and Finish Group report to the nursing and midwifery professional advisory board

Kirk, M., Tonkin, E. and Skirton, H., 2014. An iterative consensus-building approach to revising a genetics/genomics competency framework for nurse education in the UK. *Journal of Advanced Nursing*, 70(2), pp.405–420.

Kleinberger, J.W. and Pollin, T.I., 2015. Undiagnosed MODY: time for action. *Current Diabetes Reports*, 15, pp.1–11.

Lea, D.H., Skirton, H., Read, C.Y. and Williams, J.K., 2011. Implications for educating the next generation of nurses on genetics and genomics in the 21st century. *Journal of Nursing Scholarship*, 43(1), pp.3–12.

Liu, C., Ran, R., Li, X., Liu, G., Xie, X. and Li, J., 2022. Genetic variants associated with chronic obstructive pulmonary disease risk: cumulative epidemiological evidence from meta-analyses and genome-wide association studies. *Canadian Respiratory Journal*, 2022(1), 3982335.

Livingston, G., Huntley, J., Liu, K.Y., Costafreda, S.G., Selbæk, G., Alladi, S., Ames, D., Banerjee, S., Burns, A., Brayne, C. and Fox, N.C., 2024. Dementia prevention, intervention, and care: 2024 report of the Lancet standing Commission. *The Lancet*, 404(10452), pp.572–628.

Lopes-Júnior, L.C., Bomfim, E. and Flória-Santos, M., 2022. Genetics and genomics teaching in nursing programs in a Latin American Country. *Journal of Personalized Medicine*, 12(7), p.1128.

Magalhães-Barbosa, M.C.D., Prata-Barbosa, A. and Cunha, A.J.L.A.D., 2022. Toxic stress, epigenetics and child development. *Jornal de Pediatria*, 98, pp.13–18.

Mathis, H.C., 2022. Reducing the intimidation factor of teaching genetics and genomics in nursing. *Journal of Nursing Education*, 61(5), pp.261–263.

Matthews-Juarez, P. and Juarez, P.D., 2011. Cultural competency, human genomics, and the elimination of health disparities. *Social Work in Public Health*, 26(4), pp.349–365.

MD CALC, 2024. Simon Broome Diagnostic criteria for familial hypercholesterolaemia (FH). https://www.mdcalc.com/calc/3817/simon-broome-diagnostic-criteria-familial-hypercholesterolemia-fh (accessed 29 January 2025).

Ned, R.M. and Sijbrands, E.J., 2011. Cascade screening for familial hypercholesterolemia (FH). *PLoS Currents*, 3, p.RRN1238.

NHS, 2021. When you'll be invited for breast screening and who should go. https://www.nhs.uk/conditions/breast-screening-mammogram/when-youll-be-invited-and-who-should-go/ (accessed 21 January 2025).

NHS, 2022. NHS stop smoking services help you quit. https://www.nhs.uk/live-well/quit-smoking/nhs-stop-smoking-services-help-you-quit/ (accessed 29 January 2025).

NHS England, 2022. Accelerating genomic medicine in the NHS. https://www.england.nhs.uk/long-read/accelerating-genomic-medicine-in-the-nhs/ (accessed 29 May 2025).

NHS England, 2024. The NHS Jewish BRCA Testing Programme. https://jewishbrca.org/

NHS England, 2025. National Genomic Test Directory: Rare and inherited disease eligibility criteria. https://www.england.nhs.uk/wp-content/uploads/2025/01/rare-and-inherited-disease-eligibility-criteria-V7.1-OFFICIAL-2.pdf (accessed 24 January 2025).

NHS England, 2023. The 2023 genomic competency framework for UK nurses. https://www.genomicseducation.hee.nhs.uk/wp-content/uploads/2023/12/2023-Genomic-Competency-Framework-for-UK-Nurses.pdf (accessed 29 May 2025).

NMC, 2018. *Standards of proficiency for registered nurses*. NMC, London. https://www.nmc.org.uk/standards/standards-for-nurses/standards-of-proficiency-for-registered-nurses/ (accessed 29 May 2025).

North East and Yorkshire Genomic Medicine Service, 2023. Niche 2 necessity: circle of life. https://ney-genomics.org.uk/niche-2-necessity-circle-of-life/ (accessed 5 February 2025).

Oniya, O., Neves, K., Ahmed, B. and Konje, J.C., 2019. A review of the reproductive consequences of consanguinity. *European Journal of Obstetrics & Gynecology and Reproductive Biology*, 232, pp.87–96.

Orringer, 2018. Inside the Angelina Jolie effect on breast reconstruction. https://www.plasticsurgery.org/news/blog/inside-the-angelina-jolie-effect-on-breast-reconstruction (accessed 24 January 2025).

Prasad, C., Imrhan, V. and Rew, M., 2011. Introducing nutritional genomics teaching in undergraduate dietetic curricula. *Journal of Nutrigenetics and Nutrigenomics*, 4(3), pp.165–172.

Primary Care Genetics, 2017. Red flags for clinical practice. https://www.primarycaregenetics.org/ (accessed 29 January 2025).

Pursnani, S. and Merchant, M., 2020. South Asian ethnicity as a risk factor for coronary heart disease. *Atherosclerosis*, 315, pp.126–130.

Rahma, A.T., Elsheik, M., Ali, B.R., Elbarazi, I., Patrinos, G.P., Ahmed, L.A. and Al Maskari, F., 2020. Knowledge, attitudes, and perceived barriers toward genetic testing and pharmacogenomics among healthcare workers in the United Arab Emirates: a cross-sectional study. *Journal of Personalized Medicine*, *10*(4), p.216.

Read, C.Y. and Ward, L.D., 2018. Misconceptions about genomics among nursing faculty and students. *Nurse Educator*, *43*(4), pp.196–200.

Shepherd, M., Colclough, K., Ellard, S. and Hattersley, A.T., 2014. Ten years of the national genetic diabetes nurse network: a model for the translation of genetic information into clinical care. *Clinical Medicine*, 14(2), p.117.

Tonkin, E. and Skirton, H., 2013. The role of genetic/genomic factors in health, illness and care provision. *Nursing Standard (through 2013)*, 28(12), p.39.

Wright, H., Zhao, L., Birks, M. and Mills, J., 2019. Genomic literacy of registered nurses and midwives in Australia: a cross-sectional survey. *Journal of Nursing Scholarship*, *51*(1), pp.40–49.

Youssef, E., Buck, J. and Wright, D., 2020. Understanding pharmacogenomic testing and its role in medicine prescribing. *Nursing Standard*, *35*(7), pp.55–60.

Genomics nursing in specialist areas

Chapter outline

This chapter focuses on specialist areas of nursing practice and the provision of care related to areas of genomic risk and of care following the diagnosis of genetic conditions. It explores some of the specialist nursing skills and knowledge which are necessary to provide effective care within genomics services.

Introduction

Working as a part of multidisciplinary teams, nurses have the most contact with patients and perform many essential roles within their care. In some areas, nurses have the specialist skills and knowledge to care for patients undergoing testing and ongoing treatment for genetic and genomic conditions and appropriate nursing support can lead to their improved health outcomes (Calzone et al., 2010). The nursing community must provide the most effective care possible by using the services and technologies available and nursing roles in many settings will continue to develop and adapt as new genomics technology and treatments are discovered.

Chapter 3 explored a range of genomics practice competencies useful for all nurses. This chapter considers the skills necessary to care for and to support patients and families accessing genomics related care. Screening in response to the identification of genomic risk, testing to inform diagnosis of diseases with a suspected genomic cause and the provision of continuing care, including safe and effective treatment choices using information about a person's genotype, is becoming routine practice (Read and Ward, 2018). Specialist genomics nursing skills include advanced communication skills for giving detailed and evidence-based information about risk, testing and treatment but also for eliciting information from patients about what is important to them to help them to make decisions about their care.

DOI: 10.4324/9781003453048-4

> ### ⚕ Summary of specialist skills for genomics nursing
>
> - Facilitating population level screening
> - Facilitating access to services and health equality
> - Promoting health
> - Recording a family health history
> - Identifying risk
> - Discussing level of risk
> - Discussing the benefits and limitations of testing
> - Genetic counselling regarding the implications of testing for patients and families
> - Obtaining informed consent
> - Obtaining biological samples
> - Accessing the National Genomic Test Directory and requesting appropriate tests
> - Interpreting genomic test results
> - Sharing test results with patients
> - Requesting other investigative tests to inform diagnosis
> - Working as part of a multi-disciplinary team
> - Supporting patients and parents to receive diagnoses
> - Giving information effectively regarding genetic conditions and ongoing care
> - Linking patients and parents with ongoing psychological support
> - Signposting to other appropriate services
> - Sharing information effectively with other services
> - Discussing reproductive options
> - Discussing sharing genetic health information within families
> - Advocating for individual patients and patient groups
> - Requesting pharmacogenomic tests when required
> - Supporting patients through treatment, including administration and monitoring the effects of treatment and managing treatment side effects
> - Providing safety information and a point of contact
> - Facilitating patient enrolment in research and sharing their genomic data where appropriate
> - Cascade testing of families including obtaining individual informed consent for each test.

Recording a family health history

Relating their family history to a health professional is the first stage of the genomic testing process for many people. This history can provide the information necessary for nurses to identify potential genomic risks and to discuss next steps. A family health history may be taken at an appointment related to another episode of care or patients may present specifically to discuss their family's health history because they would like to find out whether they are at risk of inheriting a specific condition. If a risk is identified, people may be referred to speciality genomic services where their family health history can be explored in more depth by using a diagram to chart specific details. A family history, or family tree (sometimes called a 'pedigree') can help to illustrate the inheritance patterns of different phenotypes within a family. Such diagrams place the patient within the context of their whole family to explore possible genetic determinants of their health. In addition to specific conditions or events, it is useful to record the ancestry and ages of death of relatives if known.

Charting an accurate and detailed three or sometimes four generation family history can help to identify any genetic risk to a specific individual and to other family members and inform targeted health promotion, genetic screening and further tests if indicated. For example, serious cardiac events within a family, especially those occurring in people at a young age might precipitate cardiovascular health assessments for other family members. Nursing care in the first instance, following identification of increased risk, might include giving information about specific risk factors in combination with education or advice regarding diet, exercise, alcohol consumption and smoking. Nurses may also initiate cholesterol checks or other investigative tests and outline the early warning signs of disease (Lea et al., 2011).

📖 Learning activity

- Look through the resources within the Genomics Education Programme and watch the videos on recording a family health history.
- Haemochromatosis is a condition inherited in an autosomal recessive pattern which causes iron to accumulate in the body. An excess of iron can cause damage to organs and joints over time but is usually treated by venesection or chelation therapy (NHS, 2023). Using the following case study, construct a multigenerational family health history to trace the inheritance of a genetic variant which causes haemochromatosis.

Mary Smith is 55 and she is married to John Smith, 54. They are both unaffected. They have twin daughters aged 30, Emily (married to Tom) Simmons and Ruth Smith (not married). Both sisters have haemochromatosis.

Marys' mother and father (Sid and Victoria Clarke, both aged 80) and her maternal grandparents (Joan and Ian Carroll, both deceased) are/were unaffected. Mary's paternal grandfather, Rowan Clarke, and grandmother, Ivy, (both deceased) were not affected by haemochromatosis but her great grandfather Ivan Clarke (Rowan's father, deceased) had the condition. Ivan was adopted and his birth parents are not traceable. Ivan's wife, Jean, was unaffected. Jean experienced a stroke aged 77 and died shortly after.

Neither of John's parents (Clive and Margaret Smith, aged 75 and 78 respectively) are affected but Margaret's mother (John's maternal grandmother) Rita Scannell, married to Arthur Scannell (both now deceased), and Rita's sister, Eve Porter (not married, died at 'a young age' but the exact year is not known) both had the condition. Rita and Eve emigrated to the UK from Canada in the 1960s and their ancestry is Canadian, but no further details are known. Clive Smith has type 2 diabetes and Margaret Smith has chronic obstructive pulmonary disease.

Taking and drawing a family history (https://www.genomicseducation.hee.nhs.uk/taking-and-drawing-a-family-history/)

(This learning activity is linked to NHS England (2023) genomic nursing competency 1.)

Challenges to constructing a comprehensive and accurate family health history often include patients' limited knowledge of health conditions within their families beyond those affecting first-degree relatives. There is usually also less accuracy in information concerning mental health conditions, of which the relevant details are less likely to have been shared. However, extraneous detail from discussion can be useful to the health care practitioner recording a family history in terms of any contributory environmental and lifestyle risks mentioned by the patient (Lea et al., 2011).

Genetic counselling

For many years, suitably trained nurses have provided genetic counselling and in the US some nursing roles, for example in oncology settings, are fulfilled by nurse genetic counsellors (Lea and Monsen, 2003). In the UK, there is more separation between the two roles, but some genetic counsellors are also registered nurses, and some registered nurses provide genetic counselling within their roles. Nurses working in genomics services often develop counselling skills including the ability to support patients with strategies for sharing sensitive information within their families (Tluczek et al., 2019). Nurses who are not trained to perform genetic counselling can refer to specialist genetic counsellors to manage issues outside the scope of their practice, including comprehensive discussion regarding the possible implications of genomic tests and reproductive advice.

Genetic counselling may be required at multiple stages of the patient journey and may include taking a more detailed family history. Genetic counsellors can discuss testing options in depth and establish what the patient hopes to gain from their test results. Discussion exploring patient values and priorities demonstrates respect for their autonomy and empowers people to make decisions about testing which are right for them. Next steps might include the sharing of results within families and supporting first-degree relatives to book a consultation with the most appropriate practitioner or service where, if the patient consents, they will be able to access index testing records using a unique identification code.

For non-invasive pre-natal testing – genomic testing performed during pregnancy – genetic counsellors will go on to support prospective parents to receive their results and to discuss appropriate next steps regarding the continuation of pregnancies and future reproductive planning. When receiving a neonatal diagnosis, genetic counselling will also help parents to predict how an inherited condition may affect future pregnancies. In some cases, testing a previous baby's stored blood spots (from routine heel prick tests for phenylketonuria, thalassaemia, haemophilia and primary haemochromatosis) may provide further information about the parents' risk of having another baby with the same condition in the future. This may also lead to the offer of cascade tests for other family members to find out if they have the condition.

🔍 Case study

Colin is 60 and has just become a grandfather. His father died at a young age (52) of an unknown cause and over the past six months or so, Colin has developed some symptoms which are significantly impacting on his life. Colin has been a keen gardener up until now, but he has had a gradually increased swelling in his ankles and some shortness of breath. Fatigue is also limiting how much he can do in a day. Colin sometimes has palpitations which make him very anxious.

Colin's GP thinks that these symptoms might indicate dilated cardiomyopathy or a similar condition and Colin is referred to a nurse led clinic at his regional clinical genetics service for diagnostic tests. When he attends for his appointment, the Clinical Nurse Specialist asks Colin if he is happy to have a detailed discussion about genomics. She provides a private room where they discuss pathogenic (disease-causing) genetic variants as a possible cause for Colin's symptoms and the possible implications of this for Colin and his family.

The information he gives determines that in addition to other investigations, a genomic test would be beneficial, and that Colin meets the criteria in the National Genomic Test Directory (NGTD) for a cardiac panel test. The clinical nurse specialist (CNS) is careful to make clear that the test results might take a long time to be returned and might not provide a clear answer; it's possible that the cause of the condition might not be genetic or that tests identify a rare or unique genetic cause, leading to no other helpful information.

Colin really wants to identify the cause of his symptoms for himself and his family – his daughter Lauren has just had her first baby. The CNS says she will refer Colin to a genetic counsellor. There are some cardiac events in Colin's family health history and if his test results show an inherited variant linked to a specific a heart condition, the history indicates relatives who may also carry this variant. The genetic counsellor can facilitate the sharing of information within Colin's family and referring those at risk for predictive genetic testing.

In 8 weeks, when Colin's test results come back from the lab, the CNS interprets the report. The result given states that a variant of uncertain significance has been identified, which is disappointing news for Colin. The CNS explains that there is no empirical evidence of a likely prognosis for people with this variant and that the variant may be unique to Colin's family.

The CNS goes on to discuss Colin's case at the next multi-disciplinary team meeting. Some measures can be taken to manage Colin's symptoms, but more information is needed to structure his ongoing care. The consultant suggests a family study or segregation analysis of Colin's family tree to learn more about the identified variant, including how much it may be contributing to Colin's symptoms, and information to help predict its inheritance pattern.

After a few weeks, Colin returns to the genetic counsellor for further discussion to help him understand how he feels about the test result. He is experiencing low mood, and she decides to refer him to a mental health service for further support.

Obtaining consent for genomic testing

Owing to the number of points for discussion, ensuring that a patient has had adequate preparation to provide informed consent for a genomic test can be a lengthy and involved process becoming more complex if ethical concerns are identified. Ethical issues may be related to a person's capacity to provide consent or to the sharing of information about risks to the health of another family member. Maintaining patient privacy and confidentiality and managing a lack of capacity to consent are discussed in Chapter 6. Key points for discussion include the specific tests requested and the implications of any results. Patients can be reassured at this time that their test results will remain confidential unless they wish to share them. Some patients may wish to know what will happen to any biological samples provided after the test has taken place.

Limitations to the genomic testing process should be highlighted to manage patient expectations. For example, a 'normal' result does not necessarily mean that a person's condition is not genetic in origin; what we know changes as genomic science develops and many presentations may not have been previously identified or linked to existing named conditions. Genomics nurses and genetic counsellors must ensure that patients understand the significance of any potential results for them and for their family members. This includes both results concerning a particular condition and incidental findings. The specific results a patient wishes to receive and any findings they do not wish to be informed about, regarding other possible variants or likely future health conditions, should be recorded in advance of tests. Patients should also be prompted to think about which information they might prefer to share or prefer not to share, with whom they may wish to share it and the approach they might take. Further information about obtaining informed consent for a genomic test can also be found in Chapter 6.

Requesting a test

The process of requesting a genetic test requires some knowledge about which tests are available and about the national testing infrastructure. The NGTD contains a list of tests and patient eligibility criteria. Patients should be made aware of both estimated wait times for results and how they will receive their results. The patient's GP may also be informed if the patient agrees.

📖 **Learning activity**

- Have a look at the forms (https://www.england.nhs.uk/genomics/genom-res/) used to request some of the different genomic tests available.

Giving genomic information effectively

When requesting a genomic test for an individual, nurses must provide them with information about living with the condition being tested for and all possible connotations for them if the result is positive. It may be necessary to check whether they would like to have this conversation in English, or if an interpreter is needed. Information given to patients should be comprehensive and clear and accessible to the individual. This can be achieved by using appropriate, non-clinical language and other appropriate methods, such as diagrams or pictures, to help people understand. People with an intellectual disability may have a preferred personalised communication strategy and it is important to find out what this is. When making difficult decisions, a decision aid can help to present the factors involved in each option more clearly.

Sensitivity is a vital skill. Many individuals can face challenges obtaining family health details if they are adopted or estranged, or when a parent has died at a young age, and compassion and empathy can make a difference to any emotional distress this may cause. Sensitivity when discussing cultural practices such as consanguinity or cousin marriage in relation to increased genetic risk can help to avoid patients feeling that they are being judged. Genomics nurses rely on highly developed communication skills to provide appropriate emotional support when it is needed.

A patient's needs at the point of requesting a test may be very different from those indicated when receiving a diagnosis. Genomic medicine can often appear 'test focused', but it is important to remember that while waiting for results, people may be experiencing other challenges associated with daily life. Concurrent external stressors such as moving house, relationship issues, study, work or financial stress can exacerbate patient anxiety. Everybody's experience is different, and it is important for nurses to understand individual patient experiences in order to meet their needs. Some patients can wait a long time for results that do not identify the cause of a health condition and a lack of progress towards receiving a diagnosis can cause people to feel frustrated or let down.

The information and emotional support required may change over time in relation to a person's ongoing care. Nurses often have regular contact and develop intimate knowledge about patients, their families and their lives within their communities, and this position can help them to form effective professional relationships. Trusting relationships between nurses and families can enable open communication and reduce anxiety when making difficult decisions or receiving difficult diagnoses (Calzone et al., 2010). Receiving a genetic or genomic diagnosis can affect individuals and their families in many ways, ranging from psychosocial impact to anxiety about their financial situation. Parents of children with new diagnoses may struggle to understand or accept new information and nurses may be required to clarify key facts and direct people to other sources of reliable information.

Communication between health care practitioners is different from that which takes place between health care practitioners and patients and usually includes more clinical terminology. In genomics, a condition may have multiple sub-types or presentations caused by different genetic variants and to avoid miscommunication, nurses can use a standardised vocabulary to discuss tests, test results and diagnosis. The Human Phenotype Ontology, established in June 2022 (The Jackson Laboratory, 2022), lists the agreed terms for describing specific genetic abnormalities. This helps the whole health care team to understand which conditions are suspected, exactly which tests should be ordered and the subsequent results. Terms within this ontology describe specific phenotypic abnormalities and outline the criteria which must be met in order to diagnose a specific condition.

📖 Learning activity

- Visit the Human Phenotype Ontology (https://hpo.jax.org/) website and search for 'Marfan Syndrome'.
- Look at the terms used for some of the symptoms associated with Marfan syndrome and their definitions.

Interpreting genomic test results

Specialist nurses may be required to interpret genomic test results, share information with patients and initiate appropriate actions regarding treatment or onward referral as part of their roles. It may also be necessary to outline what results may mean for patients in terms of ongoing care, and it is important to be transparent regarding any uncertainty to avoid misconceptions. Test results as they are reported may be difficult for patients or parents to understand, particularly in relation to certain conditions, and people may need help. For example, more than 100 epilepsy-causing gene variants are now understood to contribute to epilepsy or recurrent unprovoked seizures. Genetic testing for epilepsy is now more effective in reaching an accurate diagnosis and multi-gene panel tests can give enhanced information about associated risks such as developmental delay and inform decisions about seizure control. Epilepsies appearing in childhood are often accompanied by neurodevelopmental disorders including autism spectrum disorder, which may also have a genetic cause and so test results are often complex and must be read and translated by a competent practitioner to avoid any misinterpretation (Smith et al., 2023).

🩺 Skills focus – Returning genomic results

- Check the patient's records to determine which stage of their genomics journey they have reached and the information they have been given in preparation for the test results.
- Interpret the result and what it means for the patient and their family in terms of other tests or ongoing care.
- Seek support to clarify a result, if necessary, for example from your local genomics laboratory hub.
- Arrange a place and time to give the results that is appropriate for the patient – this could be at an online or a face-to-face appointment. Other specialists may also be invited if indicated.
- Communicate the result to the patient in a way that they can understand and explain the result in the context of their symptoms. Explain any predictable outcomes or uncertainties associated with the result and what this means in terms of any ongoing care.
- Check the patient's understanding of the information given, listen to any immediate concerns and offer clarity or reassurance where possible in terms of future contact and support.
- Confirm the inheritance pattern of the condition or variant if indicated and identify other members of their family who are at increased risk and should be notified of the result.
- Discuss next steps and agree a plan – this might be related to confirming a suspected diagnosis based on test results, treatment, or referral to other health professionals. It might be relevant to discuss the patient's preferences for sharing information here, for example with their GP.
- Record the points discussed in the relevant records, including important notes on mental health, cultural, religious or familial values, and any reproductive concerns raised.
- Give the patient relevant supporting information – this could include links to resources about a specific condition or information about support groups.

(Adapted from Health Education England, 2021.)

> ### ✎ General genetic test results laboratory reporting format
>
> - ■ The intended recipient of the report, usually the referring clinician.
> - ■ The name of the laboratory issuing the report.
> - ■ At least two patient and sample identifiers (e.g. name/date of birth/NHS number).
> - ■ The test results and an interpretation (using correct and appropriate nomenclature):
>   - ■ what the test was for;
>   - ■ if there is a genetic variant (or change) present in the sample DNA;
>   - ■ a description of the abnormality;
>   - ■ the location of the DNA change (which gene), including the specific implicated nucleotides (DNA sequence) and the specific amino acid (protein chain);
>   - ■ whether the variant is listed (linked to any known conditions or syndromes);
>   - ■ whether the variant can be classified as pathogenic or benign (according to the American College of Medical Genetics guidelines for germline variant classification);
>   - ■ the clinical interpretation of the result (including variants of uncertain significance);
>   - ■ any clinical information taken into account within the interpretation of results (ethnic background, genetic sex, relation of patient to an index case, clinical red flags);
>   - ■ carrier status in pre-natal samples;
>   - ■ any secondary findings;
>   - ■ any recommended family studies (if the variant is identified as a germline variant rather than a somatic or acquired variant);
>   - ■ any further recommended tests; and
>   - ■ whether a referral for genetic counselling should be made.
>
> (Adapted from Association for Clinical Genetic Science, 2020.)

Next steps

Following receipt of genetic or genomic test results or a diagnosis, nurses may collaborate with patients or parents to help structure continuing care. This may include the provision of education, organising subsequent appointments for treatment or review, or signposting people to support networks. It is often valuable for patients to be given information about local or national support groups who can provide additional benefits. The Understanding Real Life Genetics website (www.tellingstories.nhs.uk) contains over 100 real-life stories spanning the experiences of people with genetic conditions, at risk of inheriting a genetic condition or providing care for somebody with a genetic condition. This is a useful resource for nurses to learn about care needs and some of the challenges people may face in relation to living with genetic conditions. Elements of the stories told have been mapped to relevant genomic nursing competencies to enable reflection on the skills required to support people and any required self-development (Kirk et al., 2014).

The ability to attribute health problems and symptoms to a specific condition and to access specific information may provide some relief, especially following a long period of investigation or uncertainty. However, the impact of a diagnosis on an individual's mental health is something nurses may have to help them to manage. Being told that they have a genetic condition can cause a person anxiety regarding their future and affect their self-esteem or body image. There may also be associated legal, social and ethical issues around testing or results which are causing concern, for example, stigma associated with some conditions, or financial concerns including their potential inability to work or effects on health insurance, in some countries. Anxiety related to these issues can be exacerbated through a lack of information or understanding and it is useful for genomics nurses to know where to access accurate and accessible information or other sources of support which can be shared with patients facing such challenges.

💬 Support groups

- *Contact* is a charity supporting UK families by providing an A–Z directory of many genetic conditions and the full contact details of relevant support groups: https://contact.org.uk/conditions/
- *Antenatal Results & Choices* provides information and support to parents before, during and after antenatal screening: https://www.arc-uk.org/
- *Plasma of Hope* is a new charity, based in Walsall, which helps those suffering with sickle cell disease: https://plasmaofhope.org/
- *Genetic Alliance UK* provides support for those living with a genetic condition: https://geneticalliance.org.uk/support-and-information/living-with-a-genetic-rare-or-undiagnosed-condition/
- *Chromosome Disorder Outreach* is an American educational website which contains links to chromosomal disorder specific support groups: https://chromodisorder.org/
- *Unique* is an international charity for anyone affected by rare chromosomal and gene disorders: https://rarechromo.org/

Treatment

Advances in nursing care include supporting those receiving recently developed or newly licensed treatments, for example monoclonal antibodies or gene therapy. Nurse prescribers may be part of treatment planning and prescribing and must be skilled in the interpretation of clinical information and application to care. Monoclonal antibodies are a type of immunotherapy which uses a patient's own immune system to fight some types of cancer through recognition and binding to antigens on the surface of cancer cells. Monoclonal antibodies have been developed for lots of different types of cancer with different antigens, such as herceptin which can be used to treat breast, oesophageal and advanced stomach cancers (Cancer Research UK, 2021).

Many nurses care for patients receiving targeted treatment, particularly in the oncology setting, and to fulfil this role effectively they must understand key pharmacological principles. Understanding the intended effects of a drug and how these effects are exerted can inform effective monitoring. Following the administration of any medication, nurses must determine whether treatment is exerting a therapeutic effect and identify and act to reduce harm from any unintended or side effects (Calzone et al., 2010). Nurses can advocate for patients and initiate discussion regarding other options if a treatment is not achieving its desired effect. They may also be involved in requesting pharmacogenomic tests prior to treatment to increase medicines safety. Pharmacogenomics is concerned with individual responses to some medications based on genetic variation, including some types of chemotherapy.

Monoclonal antibodies have not been effective in treating some pancreatic cancers and in 2023 clinical trials began to test an mRNA vaccine for pancreatic ductal adeno-carcinoma, the most common type of pancreatic cancer. The treatment involves identi-fying proteins from a patient's cancer samples which trigger an immune response and using them to create a personalised vaccine (NIH, 2023). There are new treatments being developed continually and new drugs can prompt concerns regarding their safety. Another reason for nurses to understand the pharmacodynamics of available treatments is so that they can help patients to understand their options. Patients may also be wor-ried that some treatments will be invasive or that they might not work and nurses will be required to answer patient questions concerning any risks related to their medicines.

Gene therapy

The Human Genome Project, between 1990 and 2003, heralded many new possibilities for personalised and precision medicine, including gene editing technologies to enable the correction of genetic mutations (Ledford, 2016). Stem cell or somatic cell therapies use cells or tissues that have been manipulated to change their biological characteristics to treat disorders such as cancer and some infectious diseases. Single gene (monogenic) disorders, such as cystic fibrosis, sickle cell disease, haemophilia and thalassaemia, can sometimes be cured by adding a functioning gene to replace the lack of function in a faulty copy (Peddi et al., 2022). In 2024, patients in England with severe beta-thalassaemia were among the first in Europe to receive exagamglogene autotemcel, or Casgevy, a new CRISPR-based gene therapy for blood disorders (NICE, 2024). Ongoing and new research contributes to rapid advancements in this area and new treatments are being developed and becoming more widely available each year with current extensive research into gene therapy for muscular dystrophy.

CRISPR (clustered regularly interspaced short palindromic repeats) is a technology used to edit genes by using a mechanism copied from bacterial immune systems. The Cas9 enzyme is used to split the genes of viruses, but their identities are retained for future recognition (Brazil, 2024). In germline gene therapy or genome editing, gene editing tools are used to engineer the reproductive cells and modify the genome. DNA is inserted into these cells to correct genetic variants which could be inherited by future generations (Health Education England, 2023). CRISPR can potentially correct genetic mutations before an embryo is implanted using *in vitro* fertilization, for example CRISPR-Cas9 can be used to correct a mutation in the MYBPC3 gene linked to hyper-trophic cardiomyopathy (Ma et al., 2017).

Sickle cell disease

Sickle cell disease (SCD) is an autosomal recessive condition caused by a single gene mutation in the beta globin gene (HBB) called haemoglobin S. Two copies (one from each parent) of the haemoglobin S gene, must be passed on to a child for them to inherit sickle cell disease (Figure 4.1). People who carry one faulty copy of the gene have the sickle cell haemoglobin S genotype and sickle cell trait (SCT) but do not have sickle cell disease.

When they have sickle cell disease, a person's red blood cells are sickle shaped. This can cause the cells to clump together sometimes, resulting in pain and inflammation. P-Selectin is a protein released from inflamed platelets which can make them sticky and further increase the risk of blockages in the vascular system and create the potential for a

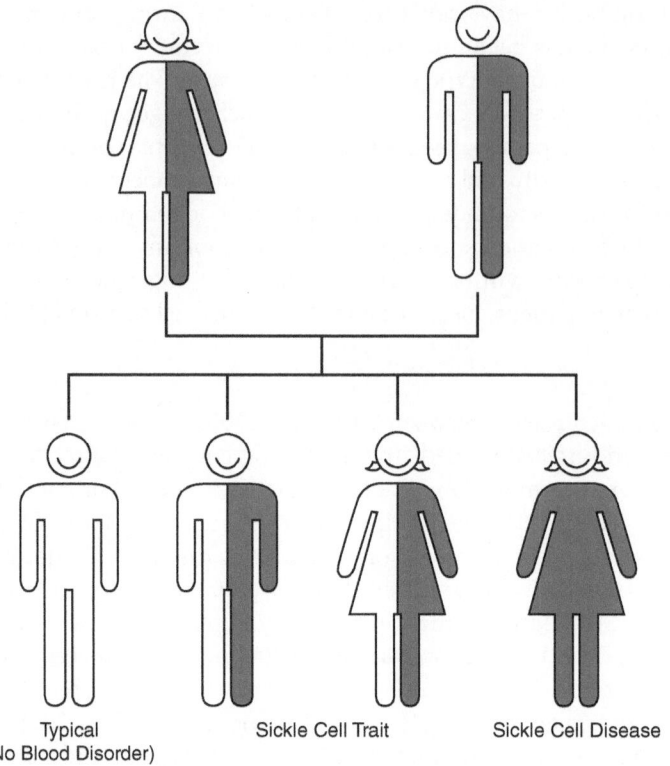

Figure 4.1 Inheritance patterns for sickle cell disease and sickle cell trait (CDC, 2024).

sickle cell crisis. Crises can occur when individuals with sickle cell disease are dehydrated, very cold or have an infection. There are multiple sickle cell phenotypes, meaning that the condition can be expressed differently in different individuals. Some people experience more pain, more severe anaemia or more crises. Disease severity can also be affected by a person's environment (including extremes of temperature) and any co-morbidities, for example those affecting the cardio-vascular system, (Karki and Kutlar, 2021).

Some medications can reduce the risk of sickle cell crisis, for example hydroxyurea, prescribed to reduce sickling in red blood cells. Sickle cell disease can lead to sickle cell anaemia through a shortage of red blood cells, which may need to be treated with blood transfusions. Casgevy is a type of CRISPR gene therapy that can be used to remove the mutation that causes sickle cell disease. Nurses may prescribe or care for patients receiving these treatments in hospital or in the community and support adherence to medication.

Nurses also have a role in educating patients about living with sickle cell disease including:

- preventing crises;
- when to seek help;
- pain management;
- managing psychological effects;
- the long-term risk of stroke and protective factors; and
- information about sickle cell disease in pregnancy and inheritance patterns.

Cystic fibrosis

Cystic fibrosis (CF) is an autosomal recessive genetic condition in which the lungs and digestive system can become clogged with thick, sticky mucus. Mutations in the cystic fibrosis transmembrane conductance regulator (CFTR) gene on chromosome 7 cause a lack of the protein responsible for transporting chloride across cell membranes. In healthy individuals, chloride can cross the membranes of secretory epithelial cells in the airways, pancreatic and biliary ducts, intestines and vas deferens. In CF, decreased chloride transport, in combination with raised intracellular sodium, and decreased extracellular water, leads to thick secretions in these areas, affecting the function of the respiratory system, the pancreas, sweat glands and the male reproductive system (Langfelder-Schwind et al., 2014). Cystic fibrosis can be diagnosed using a sweat test because the sweat of a person with CF will be low in chloride and have an increased sodium concentration.

Cystic fibrosis can cause problems with breathing and digestion from a young age. Other features include a persistent cough, which can cause the lungs to become increasingly damaged and eventually to stop working properly. People with CF may require daily chest physiotherapy at home and, depending on disease severity, they may require regular check-ups. Other contact with health providers can include hospitalisation for the administration of IV antibiotics in response to infection. Many individuals with CF lead a relatively normal life but most males will have fertility problems (Langfelder-Schwind et al., 2014).

📖 **Learning activity**

■ Search the internet to find out about common treatments for CF. You could start with NICE (https://www.nice.org.uk/guidance/ng78/resources/cystic-fibrosis-diagnosis-and-management-pdf-1837640946373).
■ Consider the nursing care patients with CF may require.
■ Many CF patients now survive into adulthood and the median predicted survival age exceeds 45 years (Férec and Scotet, 2020). Consider how changes across the lifespan might affect their needs.

Genetic testing can help to track the inheritance through a family of a disease-causing variant gene at a specific location within a chromosome. In CF, this can be done by starting with a child who has been diagnosed, looking at markers around the affected gene and trying to match these markers with a parent's genes. Understanding the path of a variant can help couples to make reproductive decisions but cannot currently be achieved as effectively in consanguineous families owing to the complex overlapping of genetic markers (Young et al., 2020).

When this diseases manifests in a child, both biological parents will either have CF or be unaffected carriers of the faulty gene (a deleterious allele). When both parents are carriers but don't have the condition, each of their children has a 1 in 4 chance of being born with CF (Férec and Scotet, 2020). A diagnosis within a family with no previous cases of CF has implications for other family members, who will be offered carrier testing. CFTR modulating treatment (for example, Kaftrio) can be used in CF to increase the number of working copies of the CFTR protein, and gene editing can sometimes be used to correct the faulty gene (Cystic Fibrosis Trust, 2024).

📖 **Learning activity**

Cystic fibrosis is an autosomal recessive condition.

- Interpret the family health history below (Figure 4.2) to trace the inheritance of a genetic variant which causes cystic fibrosis.
- Consider which members of this family are likely to be carriers of cystic fibrosis.
- Think about how you would explain to the parents (Shaun and Karina) the statistical risk of their expected child, or of any future child, being born with cystic fibrosis

(This learning activity is linked to Health Education England, 2023, competency 7.)

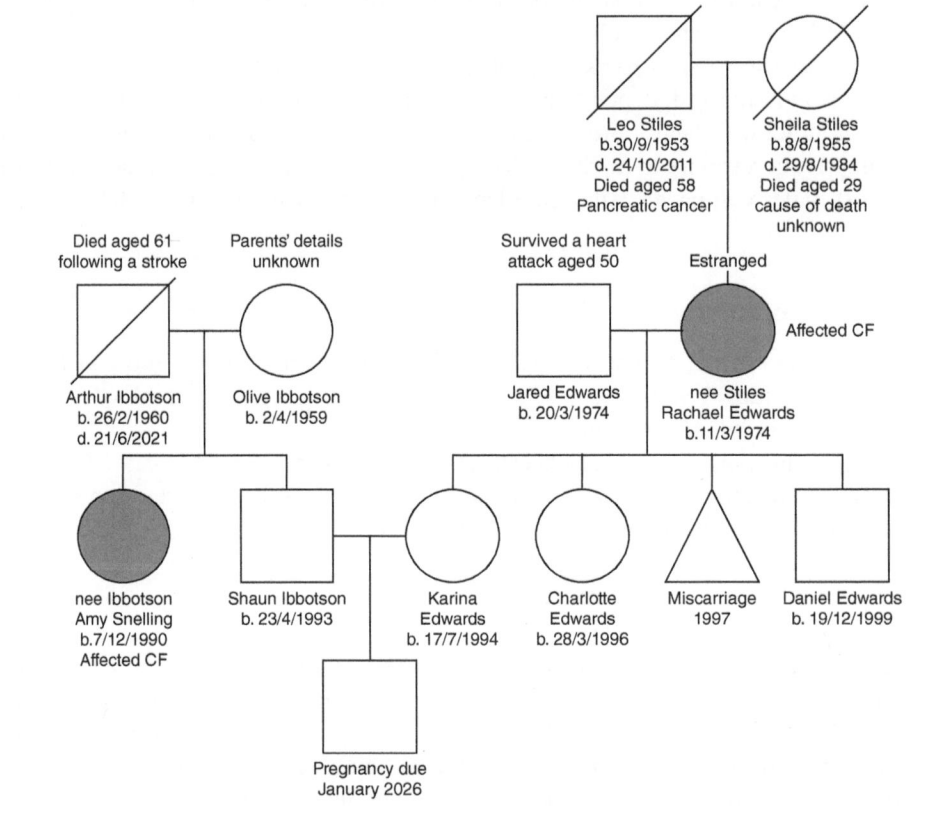

Figure 4.2 A family health history.

Carrier screening

Carrier screening can help couples to make reproductive choices prior to conception if there is a known pathogenic genetic variant within their family, for example if a parent has a biological relative(s) with cystic fibrosis. The increased risk of carrier status for specific conditions may also be linked to a person's ethnic ancestry, for example sickle cell disease which is most common in people of African descent. Expanded carrier screening can look for a specific condition and test for hundreds of other genetic disorders using the same sample. Nurses who understand basic inheritance patterns and the implications of tests for family members will know when carrier testing is appropriate and how to support patients effectively. Pre- and post-test counselling is an essential part of carrier testing to ensure that people are certain about what information they are seeking and what this information might mean for them (Rose and Wick, 2017).

Lynch syndrome

In normal physiology, mismatch repair (MMR) genes identify errors in the genetic code and try to repair them. Lynch syndrome (LS) is a pre-cancer disposition syndrome caused by inherited pathogenic variants in some high-risk mismatch repair genes, including MLH1, MSH2, MSH6, PMS2 and EPCAM. These variations lead to an increased risk of developing some cancers through unrepaired genetic errors including colorectal, skin, pancreatic, stomach, prostate, bladder and endometrial cancers (Holter et al., 2022). When people are diagnosed with colorectal or endometrial cancer, they should also be offered a test for Lynch syndrome. The test looks for DNA mismatch repair deficiency or mutations in the genes that prevent the development of these cancers. Germline testing is offered to those who test positive for LS because there are implications for their relatives. Lynch syndrome is an autosomal dominant condition and for every individual diagnosed, up to 50% of their first-degree relatives will also have LS and up to three family members will also usually be diagnosed.

Families within which LS is identified require effective nursing support, including comprehensive information about all potential outcomes and their implications to inform consent to test. This care may sometimes also require skilled management of sensitive information within families to maintain privacy and confidentiality. The high level of penetrance within families means that the condition has an increased likelihood of being passed from parent to child and so it is important to diagnose early in high-risk individuals with a history of Lynch syndrome in the family (Jasperson et al., 2010). If a patient or their partner has Lynch syndrome and they plan to start a family, *in vitro* embryos can be examined and genetically diagnosed so that only healthy ones will be implanted.

Mismatch repair deficiency cancers have a different molecular profile to non-Lynch syndrome cancers and a diagnosis of Lynch syndrome will affect a person's treatment choices, for example whether chemotherapy is indicated. Cancer genomics is changing the management of cancer for the better and Gastroenterologists can offer targeted therapies for advanced gastro-intestinal cancers caused by Lynch syndrome (Buaki-Sogo and Percival, 2022). However, part of the genomics nursing role involves managing expectations about what genomic tests can and cannot achieve. Identifying a genetic variant may not necessarily mean that a cancer can be prevented or cured but only that there may be more effective treatment options (Allen, 2021).

The NHS (2019) long-term plan for cancer aims for 75% of people with cancer to be diagnosed early and for survival rates to be increased by 5 years by 2028 (NHS, 2019). Some 95% of people who have LS don't know they have it and Lynch Nurse Educators both raise awareness and support services to integrate LS testing into mainstream medicine (Buaki-Sogo and Percival, 2022; North East and Yorkshire Genomic Medicine Service, 2024). Mainstreaming tests such as this means that people can access them locally and avoid travel costs, wait times and other barriers affecting equity of access to services across the UK.

In February 2024, a bowel cancer screening programme was launched to ensure that people aged over 25 with a diagnosis of Lynch syndrome are offered a colonoscopy every 2 years (NHS England, 2024). The prospective Lynch syndrome database contains information from carriers of MMR gene variants undergoing medical surveillance for the detection of cancers. This longitudinal cohort study aims to improve early detection, access to treatment and prognosis for LS cancers to lower recurrence rates going forward (Dominguez-Valentin et al., 2023). Other measures to reduce the risk of colorectal cancer include daily aspirin (NICE, 2020). Nurses can provide support for people with LS to make lifestyle and dietary modifications to improve outcomes. They can also initiate tests for *Helicobacter pylori*, which affects a large number of people and is known to increase the risk of stomach cancer.

Nursing care for those with inherited cardiac conditions

Inherited cardiac conditions or ICCs is an umbrella term for over 50 diseases including cardiomyopathies, aortopathies and arrhythmia syndromes. All ICCs can cause sudden cardiac death but individuals with common pathogenic genetic variants have different phenotypes and different levels of clinical risk, often making them complex and difficult to diagnose. Between 5,000 and 10,000 unexpected deaths occurring each year in the UK are caused by undiagnosed inherited diseases of the heart such as hypertrophic cardiomyopathy, dilated cardiomyopathy and congenital long QT syndrome (Alway et al., 2024).

When an individual experiences symptoms such as syncope or arrhythmia, or if there is a history of heart problems in their family, they may be referred for cardiac investigations. If they meet the eligibility criteria they may also be offered genomic testing. Specialist nurses will discuss possible outcomes with patients following a positive genomic test result, including the potential psychosocial, mental health and lifestyle impact. Some people may also be advised to avoid sport or exercise.

📖 Learning activity

GeNotes (https://genomicseducation.hee.nhs.uk/genotes/in-the-clinic/) is a useful education resource for nurses practising in some specialist areas including cardiology, oncology, primary care and paediatrics. This resource can be found within the within Genomics Education Programme and contains genomics notes for clinicians. These notes outline both 'in the clinic' scenarios to help nurses and other health care practitioners to know when they should consider genomic testing and the clinical processes for requesting tests and receiving results with practical information aligned to the National Genomic Test Directory.

■   Look at some of the scenarios in the Primary Care section (for example the presentation of a patient with a family history of cardiomyopathy, https://www.genomicseducation. hee.nhs.uk/genotes/in-the-clinic/presentation-patient-with-a-family-history-of-cardiomyopathy/) and consider the role of the nurses involved in these scenarios and the knowledge and skills they require to perform these roles effectively.

When a person is diagnosed with an ICC, their first-degree relatives can undergo predictive genomic testing. Up to 50% of family members of both sexes of families with autosomal dominant conditions will also be affected and the associated implications can cause anxiety while awaiting results, particularly in cases of sudden cardiac death. Early detection of mutations causing some inherited cardiac arrhythmias can lead to early intervention and potentially avoid complications, decrease severity and increase options for effective treatment. Some centres provide care for multi-generational ICC families led by the results of genomic tests (Alway et al., 2024). Prophylactic intervention with anti-arrhythmic drugs such as beta blockers or ACE inhibitors, prescribed for a number of known genetic mutations causing cardiac conditions, can improve outcomes. Lifestyle modifications and avoiding key risks can also be discussed, for example in Brugada syndrome avoiding a fever can reduce the risk of cardiac arrest. Defibrillators can be installed in patients' homes to increase their chances of surviving a cardiac arrest (Lea et al., 2011).

Q Case study

Morgan is 28 and plays netball for their county. They have been estranged from their family for 6 years owing to a relationship conflict. Morgan's cousin has recently been in touch to share with Morgan that his father, Morgan's uncle, has died suddenly and unexpectedly from congenital long QT syndrome. This syndrome can cause sudden death owing to altered electrical conductivity of the heart muscle (Lea et al., 2011).

On presentation at the GP surgery, the practice nurse recognises the possible genetic risks for Morgan and notes that they are very anxious. She gives Morgan some information about LQT syndrome. The practice nurse also constructs a family tree with Morgan and obtains consent to refer them to a specialist inherited cardiac conditions (ICC) nurse who she knows also practises as a genetic counsellor.

At Morgan's appointment with Stephen, the ICC nurse, the following points are discussed:

■   the genomic testing process and the time periods involved;
■   all cardiac conditions listed in the in NGTD for which Morgan is eligible to test;
■   all possible results which Morgan could receive including variants of uncertain significance
■   the benefits and limitations of testing;
■   living with the risk of sudden cardiac death should any conditions be identified;
■   potential future symptoms;
■   potential future treatments, such as beta blockers or an implantable cardioverter defibrillator;

- the potential need to avoid drugs which are known to prolong the QT interval;
- the potential risk from competitive sports;
- sharing information within the family if any conditions are identified; and
- the potential risks for any biological children Morgan may go on to have.

Morgan decides to consent for a cardiac panel test, and they agree that Stephen will contact them when he receives the laboratory results.

Paediatric nursing

Nurses support many patients and families from the early pre-testing stages of their genomics care through to requesting tests, supporting diagnosis and providing ongoing care. When nursing a baby, child, adolescent or teenager with a genetic condition, paediatric nurses perform a substantial role in their care and in their family's care. Immediately following a diagnosis, they may be required to explain inheritance patterns and to provide post-test counseling including discussion about accessing support to cope with psychosocial ramifications (Sheidley et al., 2022).

📖 **Learning activity**

- Imagine that you are supporting a family through requesting a neo-natal genomic test for a suspected chromosomal disorder.
- Make a list of skills which you think are important for sharing clinical information effectively with families. You could start by considering techniques for tailoring information to meet individual communication needs.
- Next, make a list of factors you think should be explored with this family in order to support them to decide whether to accept a test. This might include actions dependent on test results for example whether the baby's siblings should be tested to see if they are carriers for the condition.

(This learning activity is linked to NHS England (2023) genomic nursing competencies 2 and 7.)

In conditions such as Down syndrome, decreased muscle tone can affect infant feeding and cause constipation or gastro-oesophageal reflux, requiring support with digestive health and nutrition. Some conditions cause difficulty breathing and require the introduction of respiratory devices and regular assessment. Nursing care may also involve the administration of medication, monitoring the effects of medication or medication review. For those with conditions such as Duchenne muscular dystrophy and other conditions that cause muscle weakness or mobility problems, nurses may visit to help with continence care or skin integrity. School nurses support children and young people with complex health needs and with Special Educational Needs and Disabilities. Nurses must also work in collaboration with other practitioners such as occupational therapists, physiotherapists and speech therapists, necessitating the development of skills for co-ordinating care.

With regular contact, nurses can identify support needs within families and refer parents for specialist support to help manage the impact of living with a genetic condition. This might involve assessment of and discussion about any effects on mood or well-being. They can support the autonomy of adolescents with genetic conditions and to give them a voice and feelings of being in control where possible. Some conditions, including Duchenne muscular dystrophy, may be life-limiting and children and paediatric nurses in many settings, particularly hospices, must help to manage the familial implications of dying (Kirk et al., 2011).

·Ö· Reflective activity

Most people with cystic fibrosis are prescribed Creon, a pancreatic enzyme replacement therapy owing to the inability of their pancreas to produce enough enzymes. They need this to help them absorb nutrients from food.

In May 2024, a serious shortage protocol was issued for Creon® 25000 gastro resistant capsules (NHSBSA, 2024).

- Imagine you are a practice nurse to whom a patient has reported the inability to obtain this drug.
- Using Gibbs' reflective cycle (Gibbs, 1988) (Figure 4.3), consider the implications and associated feelings of those managing or affected by the shortage.

(This reflective activity is designed to support achievement of NHS England (2023) genomic nursing competency 8.)

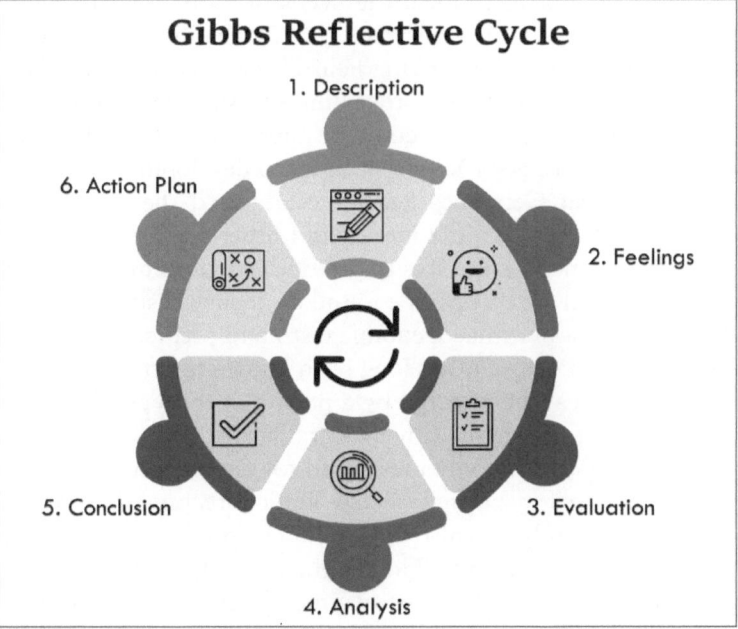

Figure 4.3 Gibbs' reflective cycle.

Specialist genomics nurses may care for people with rare diseases. Conditions are diagnosed as rare when they have not been seen before, when there is unusual presentation of a known condition or when tests show that symptoms are caused by a variant of unknown significance. A rare condition affects fewer than 1 in 2000 people and 99% of genetic conditions are classed as rare (Genetic Alliance UK, 2025). Associated symptoms can be severe and unpredictable. It can be challenging to find a molecular cause for some conditions and a whole genome approach can be effective in reaching a diagnosis. A diagnosis can have 'profound lifelong benefits' for patients and parents in terms of information, support and the ability to predict outcomes (Wright et al., 2023, p.1559).

Many patients, however, may undergo numerous tests and investigations which form part of a diagnostic odyssey where no answers are found (NHS England, 2022). Patients in this situation can access support and information from the SWAN UK (Syndromes Without a Name, https://geneticalliance.org.uk/support-and-information/swan-uk-syndromes-without-a-name/) community. Attempting to understand the experiences of those living with rare and undiagnosed conditions is vital and listening is key to supporting parents who are struggling so that targeted advice on coping mechanisms may be given. Caring for those with diagnosed or undiagnosed genetic conditions might be challenging emotionally for some nurses, who must also consider their own coping mechanisms and resilience.

Mental health

Schizophrenia often runs in families, although no single chromosomal variant which leads directly to schizophrenia has been identified. It is thought that the condition may be linked to other neurodevelopmental comorbidities such as autism, and this understanding this helps nurses to meet the needs of individuals under their care. A report by the Royal College of Psychiatrists (2023) recommends genetic testing for those with schizophrenia and co-occurring neurodevelopmental disorders. The report also recommends further research into other illnesses, such as frontotemporal or early onset (under age 55) dementia, where it could be appropriate to test for genetic variants which may have increased a person's susceptibility to developing them.

The All Wales Medical Genomics Service established the All Wales Psychiatric Genomics Service in 2022 to support nurses and other professionals involved in the care of those affected by mental illnesses to provide genetic counselling for individuals and their families. Referral criteria can be found on their website.

Nurses may also request pharmacogenomic testing to predict the safety or effectiveness of some mental health drugs. It has long been known that the therapeutic response to Alzheimer's treatment can be affected by a person's genotype (Cacabelos, 2002). It has also become apparent that many other mental health drugs such as selective serotonin re-uptake inhibitors, commonly prescribed for depression and anxiety, could be made safer through pre-treatment pharmacogenomic screening (Sreeja et al., 2024). A genome wide association study was also able to link responses to lithium, given to treat bipolar disorder with genetic variants (Hou et al., 2016). However, there is insufficient evidence to recommend screening for liver enzyme deficiencies prior to prescribing psychotropic drugs (Royal College of Psychiatrists, 2023).

Dementia is a term used to categorise conditions which cause a loss of cognitive function. These conditions are not mental illnesses but can significantly impact a person's brain functioning and impact their sense of mental health and well-being. There are different types of dementia or progressive diseases leading to cognitive decline and memory loss, including Alzheimer's and Huntington's disease. Both of these forms of dementia have genomic associations and if a person's symptoms are assessed, for example in an NHS memory clinic, following some noticeable cognitive impairment, they may be offered a genomic test. The average person's risk of developing Alzheimer's disease is 10–12%, but this risk is more than doubled if a first-degree relative has the condition. There are specific alleles associated with an increased risk of dementia and genomic tests can provide information about conditions which may occur in mid-to-later life, such as early onset Alzheimer's disease, in advance of an individual experiencing any symptoms.

In addition to their physical well-being, a person's mental health can be influenced by their genes and by environmental and lifestyle factors which can affect the genome. A healthy lifestyle has been shown to dramatically reduce the risk of developing Alzheimer's disease and nurses have an important role in helping to reduce associated risks through patient education about the risks of smoking, poor diet, lack of exercise and high alcohol intake (Dhana et al., 2020).

Awareness of genetic risk and increased awareness regarding genomic medicine means that a greater number of patients are requesting genomic tests from health services or accessing direct-to-consumer tests (Goldman et al., 2011). Receiving difficult results through either route can have a significant impact on an individual's mental health, creating a need for nursing support (Flowers et al., 2020). Variability in symptoms and age of onset and the lack of cure for some conditions means that there is little benefit in identifying genetic mutations that increase a person's risk of developing a degenerative disease but this insight may greatly increase their anxiety. Once received, test results cannot be 'taken back' and effective genetic counselling prior to testing for adult-onset conditions, especially those that usually appear in later life, can support pre-test decision making (Goldman et al., 2011, p.9).

Summary

Nurses are instrumental in the provision of effective genomics related care, including giving information, referral to other services, administering and monitoring treatment, and providing emotional support. Safe and effective care requires specialist skills and knowledge regarding genetic conditions and inheritance patterns, genomic testing and care pathways, support services and ethical and legal guidance. Effective genomics nursing care can significantly improve experiences and outcomes for patients.

Specialist education and resources for nurses

- The Medline Plus database is a useful resource for nurses. Users can search or browse information about hundreds of genetic conditions, listed alphabetically, to explore signs and symptoms, genetic causes, and inheritance patterns. Medline Plus also provides information on specific chromosomal conditions. This information is in an accessible format and suitable to share with patients: https://medlineplus.gov/genetics/condition/ https://medlineplus.gov/genetics/chromosome/

- The Genomics Education Programme includes a film series exploring the breadth of experiences of patients living with genomic conditions to help health care practitioners to understand some of the challenges: genomicseducation.hee.nhs.uk/education/videos/my-genomics-journey-three-perspectives/
- The GeneEqual Toolkit has been designed to support communication about genetics with patients with intellectual disabilities to help them discuss preferences for their care: https://www.genetics.edu.au/SitePages/Intellectual-disability-patient-communication.aspx
- A national e-learning programme has been developed to support health professionals to test patients for Lynch syndrome and to improve the early identification of colorectal and endometrial cancers: https://learninghub.nhs.uk/Catalogue/national-lynch-syndrome-project
- The University of Utah Genetic Science Learning Center is a useful resource for information about genetics, genetic conditions and gene therapy: https://learn.genetics.utah.edu/content/genetherapy/
- The National Human Genome Research Institute provides a guide to interpreting genomic test results: https://www.genome.gov/sites/default/files/media/files/2020-04/Guide_to_Interpreting_Genomic_Reports_Toolkit.pdf
- The (US) Secretary's Advisory Committee on Heritable Disorders in Newborns and Children has produced a resource for primary care nurses involved in non-invasive prenatal screening (NIPS). Follow the link to access a communication guide to help communicate positive results from newborn screening: https://www.hrsa.gov/sites/default/files/hrsa/advisory-committees/heritable-disorders/resources/achdnc-communication-guide-newborn.pdf
- The (US) Society for Women's Health Research also has information for health care practitioners navigating a positive NIPS result: https://swhr.org/considering-the-patient-experience-in-noninvasive-prenatal-screening/
- Agios is a US pharmaceutical company, and their website has information for patients about metabolic and blood disorders and rare diseases, including thalassaemia and pyruvate kinase deficiency. Some of these resources are in different languages: https://www.agios.com/patients-partners/patients-caregivers/patient-resources/
- The Genomics Education Programme GeNotes pages provide information for health care practitioners on UK clinical pathways for managing genomic conditions within different specialities, including cardiology: https://www.genomicseducation.hee.nhs.uk/genotes/cardiology/

Resources for patients
- The Seattle Children's Hospital website has information available on many genetic conditions for patients and families at a US 8th grade/UK year 9 reading level: https://www.seattlechildrens.org/conditions/a-z/
- The Genetic and Rare Diseases Information Centre has information about genetic diseases and organisations to support patients (this resource is American): https://rarediseases.info.nih.gov/
- The University of Leicester provides a series of short informative podcasts about gene mutations and cancer (including Lynch syndrome): https://le.ac.uk/vgec/topics/gene-mutations-and-cancer

- Rare Disease UK has patient empowerment group to ensure patient voices are heard in developing UK policy for those with rare diseases: https://geneticalliance. org.uk/campaigns-and-research/rare-disease-uk/

- The SPARK website contains information about sickle cell disease for patients and families. This site also has a simple to use interactive Punnett square tool for determining the genetic inheritance of sickle cell disease: https://www. sparksicklecellchange.com/sickle-cell-genetics/inheritance

- Manchester UK University NHS Foundation Trust has published multi-language patient information leaflets for rare disease patients and for cancer patients: https:// mft.nhs.uk/nwglh/documents/wgs-forms/translations-of-rare-disease-wgs-patient-information-leaflet/; https://mft.nhs.uk/nwglh/documents/wgs-forms/translations-of-cancer-wgs-patient-information-leaflet/

- Airedale NHS Foundation Trust and Bradford Teaching Hospitals NHS Foundation Trust have launched an online hub including a series of videos and written information to explain more about Lynch syndrome and how the trusts test for it: https://www.airedale-trust.nhs.uk/service/lynch-syndrome-patient-support/; https://www.bradfordhospitals.nhs.uk/lynch-syndrome-patient-support/

References

All Wales Medical Genomics Service, 2022. All Wales Psychiatric Genomics Service. https://medicalgenomicswales.co.uk/index.php/en/health-professional-information/all-wales-psychiatric-genomics-service

Allen, D., 2021. Cancer nursing and genomics. *Cancer Nursing Practice*, 20(2), pp.17–19. https://journals.rcni.com/cancer-nursing-practice/feature/cancer-nursing-and-genomics-cnp.20.2.17.s10/full

Alway, T., Bastiaenen, R., Pantazis, A., Robert, L., Akilapa, R., Whitaker, J., Page, S.P. and Carr-White, G., 2024. The development of inherited cardiac conditions services: current position and future perspectives. *British Medical Bulletin*, 150(1), pp.11–22.

Association for Clinical Genetic Science, 2020. General genetic reporting laboratory recommendations. https://www.acgs.uk.com/media/11649/acgs-general-genetic-laboratory-reporting-recommendations-2020-v1-1.pdf (accessed 31 October 2024).

Brazil, R., 2024. Targeting better safety: next steps for CRISPR therapeutics https://pharmaceutical-journal.com/article/feature/targeting-better-safety-next-steps-for-crispr-therapeutics (accessed 4 October 2024).

Buaki-Sogo, M. and Percival, N., 2022. Genomic medicine: the role of the nursing workforce. *Nursing Times*, 118, pp.1–3.

Cacabelos, R., 2002. Pharmacogenomics for the treatment of dementia, *Annals of Medicine*, 34(5), pp.357–379.

Calzone, K.A., Cashion, A., Feetham, S., Jenkins, J., Prows, C.A., Williams, J.K. and Wung, S.F., 2010. Nurses transforming health care using genetics and genomics. *Nursing Outlook*, 58(1), pp.26–35.

Cancer Research UK, 2021. Monoclonal antibodies. https://www.cancerresearchuk.org/about-cancer/treatment/targeted-cancer-drugs/types/monoclonal-antibodies (accessed 18 December 2024).

CDC, 2024. Sickle cell disease. https://www.cdc.gov/sickle-cell/sickle-cell-trait/index.html (accessed 4 March 2024).

Cystic Fibrosis Trust, 2024. CF genetic therapies. https://www.cysticfibrosis.org.uk/research/cf-genetic-therapies (accessed 17 October 2024).

Dhana, K., Evans, D.A., Rajan, K.B., Bennett, D.A. and Morris, M.C., 2020. Healthy lifestyle and the risk of Alzheimer dementia: findings from 2 longitudinal studies. *Neurology*, *95*(4), pp.e374–e383.

Dominguez-Valentin, M., Haupt, S., Seppälä, T.T., Sampson, J.R., Sunde, L., Bernstein, I., Jenkins, M.A., Engel, C., Aretz, S., Nielsen, M. and Capella, G., 2023. Mortality by age, gene and gender in carriers of pathogenic mismatch repair gene variants receiving surveillance for early cancer diagnosis and treatment: a report from the prospective Lynch syndrome database. *EClinicalMedicine*, *58*, https://doi.org/10.1016/j.eclinm.2023.101909

Férec, C. and Scotet, V., 2020. Genetics of cystic fibrosis: Basics. *Archives de Pédiatrie*, *27*, pp.eS4–eS7.

Flowers, E., Leutwyler, H. and Shim, J.K., 2020. Direct-to-consumer genomic testing: Are nurses prepared? *Nursing2023*, *50*(8), pp.48–52.

Genetic Alliance UK, 2025. Genetic rare and undiagnosed conditions explained. https://geneticalliance.org.uk/support-and-information/about-genetics/ (accessed 25 February 2025).

Gibbs, G., 1988. *Learning by Doing: a Guide to Teaching and Learning Methods*. Further Education Unit.

Goldman, J.S., Hahn, S.E., Catania, J.W., Larusse-Eckert, S., Butson, M.B., Rumbaugh, M., Strecker, M.N., Roberts, J.S., Burke, W., Mayeux, R. and Bird, T., 2011. Genetic counseling and testing for Alzheimer disease: joint practice guidelines of the American College of Medical Genetics and the National Society of Genetic Counselors. *Genetics in Medicine*, *13*(6), pp.597–605.

Health Education England, 2021. Returning genomic test results: A competency framework. https://www.genomicseducation.hee.nhs.uk/wp-content/uploads/2021/07/Returning-genomic-results-competencies-210726.pdf (accessed 8 November 2024).

Health Education England, 2023. Genomics Education Programme. What are genome editing and gene therapy? https://www.genomicseducation.hee.nhs.uk/blog/what-are-genome-editing-and-gene-therapy/ (accessed 7 November 2024).

Holter, S., Hall, M.J., Hampel, H., Jasperson, K., Kupfer, S.S., Larsen Haidle, J., Mork, M.E., Palaniapppan, S., Senter, L., Stoffel, E.M. and Weissman, S.M., 2022. Risk assessment and genetic counseling for Lynch syndrome – practice resource of the National Society of Genetic Counselors and the Collaborative Group of the Americas on Inherited Gastrointestinal Cancer. *Journal of Genetic Counseling*, *31*(3), pp.568–583.

Hou, L., Heilbronner, U., Degenhardt, F., Adli, M., Akiyama, K., Akula, N., Ardau, R., Arias, B., Backlund, L., Banzato, C.E. and Benabarre, A., 2016. Genetic variants associated with response to lithium treatment in bipolar disorder: a genome-wide association study. *The Lancet*, *387*(10023), pp.1085–1093.

Jasperson, K.W., Tuohy, T.M., Neklason, D.W. and Burt, R.W., 2010. Hereditary and familial colon cancer. *Gastroenterology*, *138*(6), pp.2044–2058.

Karki, N.R. and Kutlar, A., 2021. P-selectin blockade in the treatment of painful vaso-occlusive crises in sickle cell disease: a spotlight on crizanlizumab. *Journal of Pain Research*, pp.849–856.

Kirk, M., Campalani, S., Doris, F., Heron, J., Metcalfe, G.M.A., Patch, C. and Calzone, K., 2011. Genetics/genomics in nursing and midwifery: Task and Finish Group report to the Nursing and Midwifery Professional Advisory Board, Department of Health. https://assets.publishing.service.gov.uk/media/5a7cb326ed915d63cc65c50d/dh_131947.pdf (accessed 29 May 2025).

Kirk, M., Tonkin, E. and Skirton, H., 2014. An iterative consensus-building approach to revising a genetics/genomics competency framework for nurse education in the UK. *Journal of Advanced Nursing*, *70*(2), pp.405–420.

Langfelder-Schwind, E., Karczeski, B., Strecker, M.N., Redman, J., Sugarman, E.A., Zaleski, C., Brown, T., Keiles, S., Powers, A., Ghate, S. and Darrah, R., 2014. Molecular testing for cystic fibrosis carrier status practice guidelines: recommendations of the National Society of Genetic Counselors. *Journal of Genetic Counseling*, *23*, pp.5–15.

Lea, D.H. and Monsen, R.B., 2003. Preparing nurses for a 21st century Rolein genomics-based health Care. *Nursing Education Perspectives*, 24(2), pp.75–80.

Lea, D.H., Skirton, H., Read, C.Y. and Williams, J.K., 2011. Implications for educating the next generation of nurses on genetics and genomics in the 21st century. *Journal of Nursing Scholarship*, 43(1), pp.3–12.

Ledford, H., 2016. CRISPR: gene editing is just the beginning. *Nature*, 531(7593), pp.156–159.

Ma, H., Marti-Gutierrez, N., Park, S. W., Wu, J., Lee, Y., Suzuki, K., and Mitalipov, S., 2017. Correction of a pathogenic gene mutation in human embryos. *Nature*, 548(7668), 413–419.

NHS, 2019. Long term plan. https://www.longtermplan.nhs.uk/publication/nhs-long-term-plan/ (accessed 6 November 2024).

NHS, 2023. Haemochromatosis. https://www.nhs.uk/conditions/haemochromatosis/ (accessed 18 December 2024)

NHSBSA, 2024. SSP Creon® 25000 gastro-resistant capsules. https://www.nhsbsa.nhs.uk/sites/default/files/2024-05/Endorsement%20Guidance%20SSP061%20Creon%2025000%20restriction%20FINAL%2024052024.pdf (accessed 28 February, 2025).

NHS England, 2022. Accelerating genomic medicine in the NHS. https://www.england.nhs.uk/long-read/accelerating-genomic-medicine-in-the-nhs/ (accessed 28 August 2024).

NHS England, 2023. The 2023 Genomic Competency Framework for UK Nurses. https://www.genomicseducation.hee.nhs.uk/wp-content/uploads/2023/12/2023-Genomic-Competency-Framework-for-UK-Nurses.pdf (accessed 29 May 2025).

NHS England, 2024. News. https://www.england.nhs.uk/2024/02/thousands-with-cancer-causing-condition-offered-life-saving-nhs-bowel-cancer-screening/ (accessed 6 November 2024).

NICE, 2020. Guideline NG151: Colorectal cancer. https://www.nice.org.uk/guidance/ng151/chapter/Recommendations#prevention-of-colorectal-cancer-in-people-with-lynch-syndrome (accessed 6 November 2024).

NICE, 2024. News. https://www.nice.org.uk/news/articles/worlds-first-gene-editing-therapy-for-blood-disorder-to-be-available-to-hundreds-of-patients-in-england (accessed 18 December 2024).

NIH, 2023. News. https://www.nih.gov/news-events/nih-research-matters/mrna-vaccine-treat-pancreatic-cancer (accessed 18 December, 2024).

North East and Yorkshire Genomic Medicine Service, 2024 Think genomics. https://ney-genomics.org.uk/wp-content/uploads/2024/07/Flashcard-AI-update.pdf England (accessed 11 October 2024).

North East and Yorkshire Genomic Medicine Service, 2023. Focus on: The Lynch Pins. https://learninghub.nhs.uk/Catalogue/national-lynch-syndrome-project (accessed 6 November 2024).

Peddi, N.C., Ramesh, H.M., Gude, S.S., Gude, S.S. and Vuppalapati, S., 2022. Intrauterine fetal gene therapy: is that the future and is that future now? *Cureus*, 14(2), https://doi.org/10.7759/cureus.22521

Read, C.Y. and Ward, L.D., 2018. Misconceptions about genomics among nursing faculty and students. *Nurse Educator*, 43(4), pp.196–200.

Rose, N.C. and Wick, M., 2018, April. Carrier screening for single gene disorders. *Seminars in Fetal and Neonatal Medicine*, 23(2), pp. 78–84.

Royal College of Psychiatrists, 2023. The role of genetic testing in mental health settings. https://www.rcpsych.ac.uk/improving-care/campaigning-for-better-mental-health-policy/college-reports/2023-college-reports/the-role-of-genetic-testing-in-mental-health-settings-(cr237) (accessed 26 February 2025).

Sheidley, B.R., Malinowski, J., Bergner, A.L., Bier, L., Gloss, D.S., Mu, W., Mulhern, M.M., Partack, E.J. and Poduri, A., 2022. Genetic testing for the epilepsies: a systematic review. *Epilepsia*, 63(2), pp.375–387.

Smith, L., Malinowski, J., Ceulemans, S., Peck, K., Walton, N., Sheidley, B.R. and Lippa, N., 2023. Genetic testing and counseling for the unexplained epilepsies: an evidence-based practice guideline of the National Society of Genetic Counselors. *Journal of Genetic Counseling*, 32(2), pp.266–280.

Sreeja, V., Jose, A., Patel, S., Menon, B., Athira, K.V. and Chakravarty, S., 2024. Pharmacogenetics of selective serotonin reuptake inhibitors (SSRI): a serotonin reuptake transporter (SERT)-based approach. *Neurochemistry International*, *173*, p.105672.

The Jackson Laboratory (2022) The Human Phenotype Ontology. https://hpo.jax.org/app/

Tluczek, A., Twal, M.E., Beamer, L.C., Burton, C.W., Darmofal, L., Kracun, M., Zanni, K.L. and Turner, M., 2019. How American nurses association code of ethics informs genetic/genomic nursing. *Nursing ethics*, *26*(5), pp.1505–1517.

Wright, C.F., Campbell, P., Eberhardt, R.Y., Aitken, S., Perrett, D., Brent, S., Danecek, P., Gardner, E.J., Chundru, V.K., Lindsay, S.J. and Andrews, K., 2023. Genomic diagnosis of rare pediatric disease in the United Kingdom and Ireland. *New England Journal of Medicine*, *388*(17), pp.1559–1571.

Young, E., Bowns, B., Gerrish, A., Parks, M., Court, S., Clokie, S., Mashayamombe-Wolfgarten, C., Hewitt, J., Williams, D., Cole, T. and Allen, S., 2020. Clinical service delivery of noninvasive prenatal diagnosis by relative haplotype dosage for single-gene disorders. *The Journal of Molecular Diagnostics*, *22*(9), pp.1151–1161.

Genomics and cancer care

Chapter outline
This chapter outlines how genomic data can underpin improved diagnosis and targeted treatment to achieve improved outcomes in cancer care. How genomics can help to support precision oncology or cancer treatment, and care planned in response to genomic information about an individual's specific type of cancer, is considered. This chapter also explores how the already significant role of the nurse in cancer care is changing and developing in line with rapid developments in genomics technology.

Introduction

Cancer is a disease of the genome which affects cell growth. It is caused by inherited variations in a person's genetic code and/or damage to single or multiple genes or spontaneous changes during cell division. Oncology is an area in which genomic testing technology and infrastructure have received extensive focus and resources to develop quickly. This is because information from the genome can enable health care practitioners to identify and treat certain cancers more effectively (Health Education England, 2019). The role of the nurse is and will continue to be central in supporting patients and families effectively through cancer and genomics-competent nurses have a pivotal role in the evolution of health care services (Calzone et al., 2010).

Inheritance and cancer

Somatic variations in specific cells are the result of epigenetic changes to the genes, acquired within an individual's lifespan, and these changes are the most common cause of cancer (Allen, 2021). Damage to the genetic material within individual cells can cause cell mutations which affect gene expression. This can be significant when certain genes are caused to be 'switched off' and not expressed when they are needed, specifically those that protect against the growth of cancer cells. Somatic changes can occur in combination with an individual's inherited pre-disposition to certain cancers and this will increase a person's risk of developing those cancers.

Specific inherited or 'germline' variations within a person's genetic code are responsible for about 5–10% of all cancers (Macmillan Cancer Support, 2023A). Some genetic variations can be pathogenic or disease causing but not everybody who inherits a genetic variation will go on to develop cancer. Genetic variations can be benign or of uncertain significance; there are many known variations to the BRCA1 gene, commonly associated with breast cancer and most of them are not harmful (Read and Ward, 2018).

A complete copy of the genome is present in almost every cell in the body so a pathogenic variant in the genetic code will also appear in every cell (Genomics England, 2023). Cancers caused by germline or inherited genetic variants occur in reproductive cells (sperm or egg cells) and can be passed on from parent to child and through generations of a family (Allen, 2021). Approximately 5% of breast cancers are inherited. Lynch syndrome is an inherited pre-cancer syndrome which can increase the risk of developing colorectal cancer and some other cancers such as ovarian cancer, endometrial cancer and stomach cancer.

Cell changes

Cancer care is an area within which it is important to understand the difference between genetics and genomics. In addition to a person's genome, within which they may inherit more than 50 identified cancer-causing genetic variations, tumours have their own genomes which contain important information about somatic (acquired or developed) changes (Fee-Schroeder and King, 2019).

Understanding pathogenesis or how disease occurs can help health care practitioners to identify risk and to screen and diagnose cancer quickly. Knowledge about how specific cancers occur can also support treatment decisions. Different types of damage to cells can cause genetic changes or mutations. A genetic mutation can be a 'mistake' (a spontaneous re-ordering, duplication, fusion or deletion of some of the protein sequence, like a typo) occurring during cell division which is then embedded in the gene and the code which that gene carries. An amplification is the repeated duplication of a particular sequence. These mutations can result in impaired cell repair and can prevent the natural death (apoptosis) of old or damaged cells (Cancer Research UK, 2023).

Spontaneous deamination is a type of mutagenesis or fault which occurs when new genes are being made which inhibits the replication of nucleotide bases. Mistakes during the copying of DNA enzymes can result in 'damaged' DNA. Chemical imbalances in the intracellular environment can also precipitate reactions at a molecular level and instigate processes that cause mutagenesis and affect cell reparation such as reactions involving water or oxygen molecules which cause oxidative and hydrolytic stress (Chatterjee and Walker, 2017).

Exogenous or environmental harm may also occur and cause alkylation or damage which prevents protein synthesis by inhibiting the transcription of DNA into RNA (Chatterjee and Walker, 2017). Cancers are more prevalent in older adults because they have experienced greater exposure to elements which cause cell damage and a reduction in cell reparation over the course of their lifetime (Cancer Research UK, 2023).

External factors which can damage cells and the genetic material within include ultra-violet light from the sun which is a form of radiation and the leading cause of some skin cancers (Primiero et al., 2022; Friend, 2022). Radon gas, air pollution, asbestos, radiation and occupational exposure to other harmful substances can all increase the risk of lung cancer. Some industrial chemicals are alkylating agents that can modify the DNA of factory workers, leading to pathogenic genetic mutations. It is well known that inhaled carcinogens such as cigarette smoke can cause cancer in the respiratory system and upper digestive tract, including the pancreas (Martin, 2020).

Carcinogens or substances which can cause physiological damage leading to cancer can also be ingested via some foods, like processed meats. This will affect cells in the gastro-intestinal tract and in the bladder as these substances are excreted in the urine. Viruses can also cause cancer. Examples include infection with the Epstein–Barr virus, human papillomavirus (HPV), hepatitis B and C, Merkel cell polyomavirus and Kaposi's sarcoma herpesvirus through which viral damage to cell DNA can promote cell carcinogenesis (Chen et al., 2014).

Environmental damage can precipitate epigenetic mutations to oncogenes, which are genes that can turn a healthy cell into a cancer cell (Snyder, 2016.) Some breast cancer tumour cells have a higher level of the HER2 (human epidermal growth factor receptor 2) protein and oncogene on the cell membrane. HER2 is an oncogene which is 'overexpressed' and 'gene amplified' in approximately 20% of breast cancers, leading to proliferation of cancer cells and preventing cancer cell death (Gutierrez and Schiff, 2011.) Damage to tumour suppressor genes (which act to control cell division, repair DNA and regulate cell death) causes them to stop functioning. Damage to these cells can also result in uncontrolled tumour growth.

Cancer and the nursing role

Nurses are at the forefront of cancer care, and many provide care within genomics-based roles and support patients through testing, diagnosis and treatment. The development of the appropriate skills and knowledge to provide a good experience within their genomics journeys for patients and their families is vital for nurses working in these specialist roles (Allen, 2021). Sound knowledge of genetics and the inheritance patterns of diseases like breast and ovarian cancer is important for nurses supporting families affected by these conditions. If a patient's presentation and a family health history of similar cancers or syndromes suggests that a person's cancer could be caused by a genetic variant, nurses can initiate the genomic testing process. Identification of specific variants means that patients can consent to nurses calculating carrier probability for family members and consulting with them to discuss testing to look for the same variant (NICE, 2023). Appropriate action can be taken to improve the outcomes of family members according to test results (Mahon, 2022). Early screening of those at increased risk of developing specific cancers can lead to early diagnosis, instigation of regular screening such as yearly colonoscopies, therapeutic intervention if indicated or even prophylactic surgery such as removal of non-essential organs at risk (Health Education England, 2019; NICE, 2023).

Genomic information is contributing to the realisation of personalised medicine and in order to provide effective care, nurses need to develop an awareness of the significance of genomics for patients and their families (Allen, 2021). However, sometimes a familial pattern of cancer may be caused by an unknown cancer gene variant for which the most effective treatment has not been recognised. This is difficult news for families to receive and nurses must feel confident to support them in this instance and to refer them for specialist counselling (Macmillan Cancer Support, 2023A).

Different cancers have different mutational signatures as a result of chromosomal rearrangements and/or gene deletions and duplications. Nurses initiating genomic tests must have sound knowledge about what is being tested for and what test results might mean for a patient. Information about a specific cancer informs diagnosis and classification of tumour subtypes. If a particular gene is damaged, genomic evidence on how the resulting cancer will behave is important for planning a patient's care with them. For example, colorectal cancers can present with increased aggressiveness and have the poorest survival times compared to other cancers.

Breast cancer and ovarian cancer

One in eight women in the UK is affected by breast cancer (Genomics England, 2023). Different types of breast cancers have specific mutations. Some breast and ovarian cancers can occur owing to long-term exposure to hormones throughout a woman's lifespan from things like contraception and hormone replacement therapy (HRT) (NICE, 2023). In these cases, when breast cancer occurs, tumours are more likely to be oestrogen and progesterone receptor positive and continued exposure to these hormones can help cancer cells to grow and spread. Tamoxifen can be used to treat breast cancer but also as a chemo-preventive drug (NICE, 2023). In 2023, the Medicines and Healthcare Products Regulatory Agency (MHRA) approved the use of anastrozole for breast cancer prevention in post-menopausal women at moderate or high risk. This hormonal treatment had previously been used outside the terms of its product licence or 'off-label' for this indication (UK Government, 2023B). This approval increases the number of options for high-risk patients.

Breast and ovarian cancers can also be caused by inherited genetic variations in three high risk genes: BRCA1, BRCA2 and PALB. These variations may be inherited in an autosomal dominant pattern. Breast and ovarian cancers are common in families where there are incidences of female breast cancer in either maternal or paternal lines. These types of cancer are more likely to be hormone receptor negative cancers where growth is not affected by oestrogen or progesterone.

The BRCA1 gene, on chromosome 17q12–21, and the BRCA2 gene on chromosome 13q12–13 are tumour suppressor genes and harmful mutations in these genes predispose 60% of women with the mutation to developing breast cancer and 15–40% to developing ovarian cancer (Lesk, 2017). Variants in these single genes have a marked effect on a woman's risk of developing cancer (Sud et al., 2023). People with Jewish ancestry are six times more likely to carry BRCA1 and BRCA2 variations and in 2024, a new national NHS Jewish BRCA testing programme was launched (NHS England, 2024).

⚙ **Thinking point**

- How do you think nurses can raise awareness of genomic risk factors in local communities?
- In what ways could nurses increase access to genomic testing for high-risk groups?

When a breast or ovarian cancer is identified in an individual, they will be offered genomic testing from a blood sample. If a specific genetic mutation is identified, discussion is initiated regarding cascade testing for their family. This is more effective when the genetic variation being looked for is known. If a germline BRCA1 or BRCA 2 pathogenic variant is not identified in genomic tests, then patients may be offered somatic testing to identify key features of the tumour and to guide treatment. However, if a variant is identified, test results can have significant implications for family members identified as carriers of the same variant. These individuals may go on to have regular screening such as mammographic surveillance, treatment such as chemoprevention or risk-reduction surgery (NICE, 2023).

Nurses can identify risk factors for BRCA gene cancers from an individual's family history (especially if there is a history of breast cancer on the maternal or paternal side), but also from other aspects of their presentation, and act quickly to improve outcomes for patients and their families.

Identifying risk

Inherited breast cancers are more likely to:

- occur bilaterally;
- occur at a young age;
- occur in conjunction with ovarian cancer;
- affect several members of the same family;
- occur in male members of an affected family (Primary Care Genetics, 2017);
- occur in those of Jewish ancestry; and
- occur in those who have had other cancers at a young age (NICE, 2023).

Variations in genes other than BRCA 1 and BRCA 2 have been identified in some familial breast cancers and research into these variants is ongoing. Research is also important for predicting prognosis for breast cancer patients (Genomics England, 2023). Nurse-led breast cancer management and counselling can alleviate symptom burden and nurses' experiences regarding the effectiveness of various interventions when caring for patients and for those at risk can contribute to health research data and to the development of clinical guidelines (Chan et al., 2020).

Nurses in all settings have an important role in health promotion and can give women information about regular and effective breast checking and how to report changes (figure 5.1). Nurses must understand their local communities and be able to care for individuals in this context. Women in ethnic minority groups are more likely to be affected by health inequalities; they may have lower levels of health literacy which can affect all aspects of cancer care from prevention to treatment and outcomes. This can affect quality of life because these women are less likely to report symptoms and changes or to give information accurately. When their needs are not met by health services some ethnic groups can be less effective at self-management than others and less adherent to treatment (Moore and Hayes, 2023).

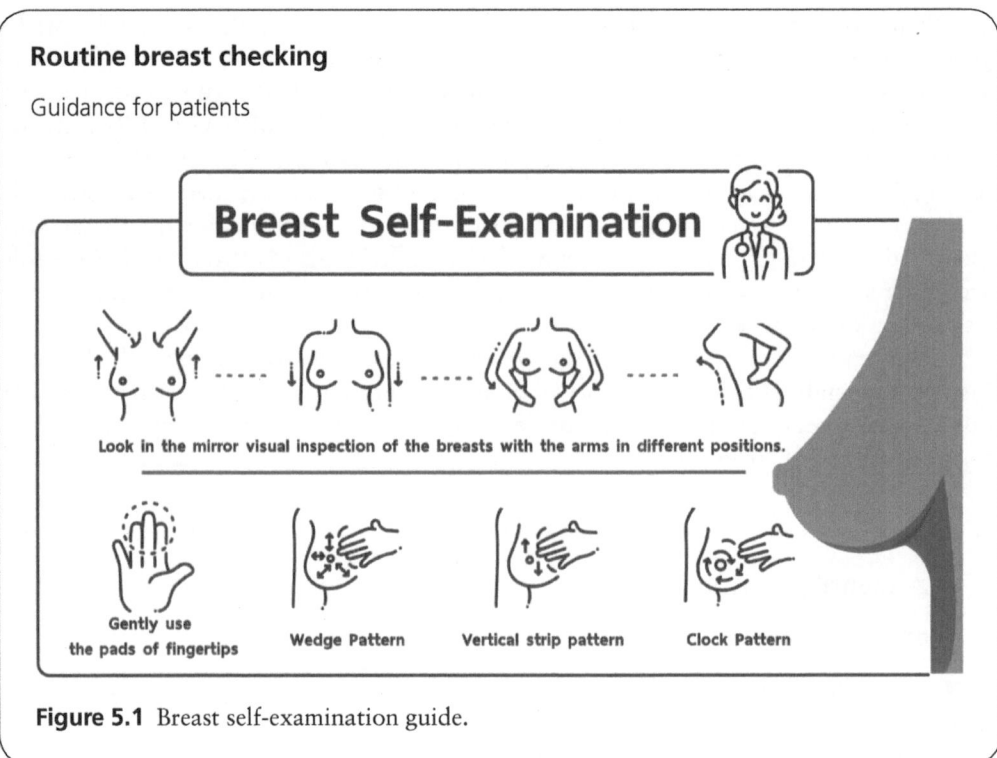

Routine breast checking

Guidance for patients

Breast Self-Examination

Look in the mirror visual inspection of the breasts with the arms in different positions.

Gently use
the pads of fingertips

Wedge Pattern

Vertical strip pattern

Clock Pattern

Figure 5.1 Breast self-examination guide.

Variation in the TP53 tumour suppressor gene, found on chromosome 17, is the most common genetic variant and can increase the risk of a number of cancers. TP53 mutations occur more frequently and more aggressively, with poorer outcomes in non-white populations. Nurses can take opportunities within routine appointments to help increase awareness of these risks and to facilitate screening opportunities (Allen, 2018).

Cancer diagnosis and targeted treatment

Chemotherapy drugs can be used in conjunction with other treatments such as radio-therapy and immunotherapy and can be very effective at treating cancer. Chemotherapy drugs may, however, not be effective in treating all metastases of a primary tumour, which may be composed of different cell types and in different locations, for example colorectal cancer can metastasize to the lungs, liver and/or peritoneum (NICE, 2021).

Many chemotherapy drugs also cause severe noxious side effects as their pharma-codynamic action at cellular targets is harmful to cancer cells and normal cells (Yang and Wang, 2018). Adverse drug reactions can be prevented by avoiding the unnec-essary prescription of chemotherapy when information from tumour DNA indicates that chemotherapy is unlikely to be effective. Sequencing DNA from a tumour and comparing this information with the sequence from healthy cells can give information about specific changes responsible for the development of a cancer (Genomics England, 2023). Analysis of somatic (acquired) variants or mutations in cancer cells is helpful when determining which treatments are likely to be effective to treat the cancer.

Accurate diagnosis and prognosis for some cancers can be informed by knowledge from the genome. Understanding of the genomics underpinning some cancers, such as the ability to identify specific characteristics or biomarkers of skin cancer, has led to significant advances in prediction. Biomarkers are important in predicting cancer behaviour and the likely effect on a patient's prognosis. Oncology nurses can look for specific genomic tumour characteristics to accelerate diagnosis, choose appropriate treatment based on the features of the tumour and improve prognosis (Friend, 2020).

In addition to a greater understanding of the causes of cancer, understanding what enables cancer cells to proliferate or spread has helped to develop effective treatments. If a particular genetic mutation is identified, patients may respond better to a cellular therapy, which works to prevent the spread instead of or in combination with traditional chemotherapy (Allen, 2021).

If a type of cancer is caused by a pathogenic inherited or germline BRCA variant, this will inform the choice of therapy and may indicate a PARP (poly-(ADP-ribose) polymerase) inhibitor as an adjuvant treatment. PARP inhibitors are effective in high genetic risk, early breast, ovarian and other gynaecological cancers in people who have a BRCA1 or BRCA2 inherited genetic mutation. These drugs can also be used in HER2 negative breast cancer and in addition to chemotherapy. They work by damaging tumour DNA and affecting the ability of cancer cells to repair damage. However, following prolonged treatment with some types of precision therapy, cancer can develop resistance resulting in disease progression (Martin, 2020). Resistance to PARP inhibitors is a common clinical characteristic for a number of tumour types (Pettitt and Lord, 2019.) This has implications for oncology nurses in terms of providing support and discussing options.

Hormone therapy such as tamoxifen may be used to target metastases of a hormone receptor-positive breast cancer. In different types of cancer, other features can determine which treatments are likely to be effective. Mutations such as HER2 amplification can be treated with Herceptin (trastuzumab), which is an HER2 monoclonal antibody that was developed to act on HER2 receptors to prevent growth and division. It also supports the immune system to attack cancer cells at tumour sites expressing HER2 (Vu and Claret, 2012).

Targeted treatments are also used treat some cancers with environmental causes. Glioblastoma is a type of brain tumour that can develop following exposure to harmful agents such as pesticides and works by altering the expression of a specific genetic protein to affect expression of the gene itself. A treatment can be given which increases survival rates by enabling cells to express a 'repair enzyme' to counteract the acquired changes in DNA and gene expression, leading to the development of a tumour (Lesk, 2017, p.289). With their extensive knowledge of gene-directed therapies, specialist oncology nurses continue to contribute to the targeted treatment of cancer (Friend, 2020).

Medicines safety

Comprehensive knowledge can support better outcomes through advanced counselling regarding risks such as the side effects associated with some treatments, which helps patients to cope and improves adherence. (NICE, 2023). Effective monitoring of medication effects and for signs of potential drug toxicity can help nurses to prevent avoidable harm (Martin, 2020). Anticipating potential drug interactions and other risks to patients being treated for cancer is another key element of medicines safety. Many drugs, including some chemotherapy drugs, must be stopped prior to the administration of immunotherapy and products such as live vaccines should not be given concurrently owing to altered immune status (Specialist Pharmacy Service, 2022).

☼ Reflection point – oncology nursing care

The nursing contribution to cancer care is unique owing to the scale and range of care needed. Nursing care is person-centred, and compassion makes a crucial difference to patients and outcomes. Cancer nurses provide advanced holistic patient support across the continuum of cancer care. They also work effectively as part of a team to communicate patient needs and coordinate care (Young et al., 2020).

- Think of some examples of actions nurses might take in an oncology setting to promote well-being in the following areas:
  - physical
  - emotional
  - psychological
  - spiritual
  - social

Pharmacogenomics and cancer treatment

Individual responses to some medicines can depend on a person's genetic makeup and information about this can help determine whether a certain medicine, including some chemotherapy drugs, will be safe for an individual. This is called pharmacogenomics. When indicated, pre-treatment screening for some cyto-toxic drugs (for example, fluoropyrimidines) prevents harm. Pharmacogenomics is explored in depth in Chapter 7. Nurses can submit information (via the yellow card biobank – https://yellowcard.mhra.gov.uk/biobank) about individual responses to medicines used to treat both somatic and germline cancers to inform research to increase medicines safety (MHRA, 2024).

Lung cancer

Lung carcinomas can be caused by alterations on specific genes, for example:

- B-Raf proto-oncogene serine/threonine-protein kinase (BRAF);
- neurotrophic receptor tyrosine kinase 1 (NTRK1);
- anaplastic lymphoma kinase (ALK);
- epidermal growth factor receptor (EGFR) (occurring more frequently in non-smokers) (Martin, 2020).

If a person is diagnosed with lung cancer, understanding the cause and nature of epigenetic cell changes can lead to more and better treatment options. Identification of individual variants directs tumour specific treatment and monitoring (Martin, 2020). Prognosis is improved when health professionals can predict the likely response of a tumour to drugs which have been developed to target specific genetic changes.

The presence of a pathogenic abnormality, such as a mutation, can be confirmed by circulating tumour DNA. This 'liquid biopsy' method is often used when tumours are deep within the lungs as it is less invasive. Blood testing can be used to detect cancer cell DNA and support diagnosis, but also to monitor treatment effects through the identification of treatment resistant mutations (Esposito et al., 2017). Tumour testing may also be achieved through biopsy. Genomic sequencing provides information on the features of individual tumours and if a variant is identified, cascade testing may be offered to family members.

The North Thames and North East and Yorkshire Genomic Medicine Services (GMSs) are collaborating in the leadership of a national pilot to integrate circulating tumour DNA testing into a routine NHS lung cancer pathway. The test, which examines tumour DNA from a blood sample, will help many people to receive earlier diagnosis and targeted treatment (North Thames GMS, 2024). The extent to which genomics benefits patients and families is manifest in the diagnosis and treatment of lung cancer and, like breast, colorectal and prostate cancer, lung cancer often runs in families. When several people within the same family inherit a cancer gene variant, this is termed familial or hereditary cancer syndrome (Macmillan Cancer Support, 2023A). Multifactorial risk factors within families, including inheritance of genetic variations plus shared environmental exposure, culture or behaviours, creates a polygenic risk or the cumulative effect of multiple factors on the phenotype. The nursing role is to both facilitate testing to identify genetic variations and to explore potentially harmful combinations with risk factors such as smoking and obesity. Recording an accurate family health history where possible and eliciting a comprehensive lifestyle history improve risk predictions and decisions regarding surveillance and care based on individual and family needs.

Cigarette smoking is the biggest risk factor for lung cancer (Martin, 2020). Many factors throughout a person's life cause epigenetic changes and increase their risk of developing lung cancer, including exposure to harmful substances from where they live, diet, smoking, second-hand smoke and/or occupational hazardous exposure. Understanding risk factors facilitates focused health promotion and support with lifestyle changes. Testing the DNA of those not yet diagnosed but at high risk can help to identify lung cancers at early stages and provide better health care, and the contribution of oncology nurses to cancer prevention and early identification is vital (Young et al., 2020).

Damage to cells from smoking can cause cancer and inherited gene variants can increase this risk. Health promotion on smoking cessation may have increased impact when supported by information about individual genetic risk. Giving and eliciting information effectively can support shared decision making and individualised planning and provide support to increase success rates (NHS, 2022).

Colorectal cancer

Approximately 30% of colorectal cancers (CRC) arise from inherited gene mutations, most commonly inherited in an autosomal dominant pattern. Some colorectal cancers develop as a result of inherited syndromes like Lynch syndrome or familial adenomatous polyposis (Jasperson et al., 2010). Lynch syndrome, explored in Chapter 4, is associated with a high risk for developing colorectal cancer and endometrial cancer and increases the risk for a number of other cancers, including stomach cancer, ovarian cancer, small bowel and pancreatic cancer (Holter et al., 2022). When somebody in the family has bowel cancer, specialist oncology nurses and genetic specialists can support families and individuals to understand their level of risk and how to manage it with actions such as regular bowel screening. When Lynch syndrome (LS) is identified as the cause of an individual's bowel cancer and their family members also test positive for LS, they can be prescribed daily aspirin to reduce their risk of developing colorectal cancer (NICE, 2021). Nurses can also help to explain options for genomic testing and manage expectations regarding all possible results, including when a variant of unknown significance or no variant is identified (Macmillan Cancer Support, 2022).

Again, the identification of specific biomarkers for somatic cancers or inherited pathogenic variants causing conditions such as LS improves the accuracy of diagnosis (NICE, 2017). Understanding the unique features of a tumour that will respond to specific therapies can determine the most effective treatment and the ability of health care practitioners to predict patient outcomes (Chung, 2022.)

DNA mismatch repair is a process through which the body keeps the genome stable when abnormalities such as deletions of base protein pairs are present. If a mismatch repair (MMR) gene is not functioning properly, owing to a known pathogenic variant that has caused damage or inactivation, this is called deficient mismatch repair activity (dMMR). MMR tumours are caused by a pathogenic variant in specific genes (MLH1, MSH2, MSH6 or PMS2 or 3′ terminal deletions of EPCAM), which can lead to microsatellite instability (MSI). Microsatellite instability is a phenotype found in tumour DNA sequences that is not present within normal cells in the same area. Microsatellite instability is a predictive biomarker identified in a significant number of colorectal and endometrial cancers and identifying whether MSI is present in solid tumours is important in the management of germline or somatic colorectal cancer (NICE, 2021).

Immunotherapy

Deficient MMR can be detected through microsatellite instability testing (Holter et al., 2022). Colon cancers with high levels of MSI have a better overall prognosis (Jasperson et al., 2010). High levels of MSI indicate that a patient will achieve a good response from immunotherapy (Martin, 2020). Immunotherapy refers to drugs that improve the body's immune response. Some types of immunotherapy block T-cell inhibition by cancer cells. T-cells are a type of lymphocyte or white blood cell which may also attack healthy cells. Checkpoint proteins can prevent T-cells from attacking healthy cells and tumours can produce checkpoint proteins to stop a patient's immune system from attacking cancer cells. The administration of drugs to stop this process (immune checkpoint inhibitors) can enhance the immune response (Robinson et al., 2023). The use of immunotherapy in place of chemotherapy can help to avoid adverse reactions from chemotherapy. The pharmacogenomic risks associated with some types of chemotherapy are explored further in Chapter 7.

Deficient MMR can also be identified through MMR immunohistochemistry testing. This test can support the identification of a genetic deficiency and in which gene it appears to guide testing for family members and speed diagnosis (Holter et al., 2022).

🔍 Case study

This fictional case study is based on guidance and a testing algorithm for Lynch syndrome in Holter et al. (2022), and has been adapted for UK nurses.

Maria is a 64-year-old, white European cis-gender female who lives in North London and works as an administrator. She sees her GP following a few episodes of bleeding per rectum. Maria is referred for an endoscopy where a colorectal tumour is identified, and a biopsy taken. Histopathology results show a CRC.

Maria is referred to her closest reference centre at St Marks Hospital and is seen by a nurse, Julie, with expertise in cancer risk assessment. St Marks is a mainstream genomic reference centre that provides genomic health care for colorectal cancer, polyposis and LS. Patients referred to this centre receive assessment, personalised advice and ongoing support from a multi-professional team (Buaki-Sogo and Percival 2022; St Mark's Hospital, 2019).

Julie performs a risk assessment for LS and offers Maria testing for this which is indicated in all cases of CRC (NICE, 2017). Lynch syndrome is an inherited, autosomal dominant condition caused by pathogenic variants in MMR genes. Julie takes Maria's family history as others in the family may be at risk of developing colorectal and other cancers if LS is diagnosed.

One of Maria's sisters, Ann, now aged 68, was treated for endometrial cancer 20 years ago. Julie recognises this as a young presentation which is a red flag for LS. No germline testing was offered at the time. Maria reports that their paternal great grandfather died at an early age, but that the cause of his death is not known.

Julie decides what tumour tests to order for Maria, who provides a blood sample. The National Genomic Test Directory lists available tests and testing criteria; tumour tests are indicated for all individuals with colorectal or endometrial cancer regardless of age (NHS England, 2022).

Maria is given the information she needs to consent to a genomic test. She records her preferences for receiving the results and signs to say she has understood the information she was given about the condition being tested for, the test and how her information will be used and stored. She also signs to say she understands the implications of all possible results. Maria consents for test results to be shared with any member of her family.

Maria is referred for genetic counselling by Julie to support discussions about the test with her family. Maria's children (two daughters) are both in their 30s and have children. Maria's brothers and sisters all also have children who may wish to start families. The sample is sent for next-generation sequencing for MSI and MMR immunohistochemistry at the nearest laboratory.

The test results take 8 weeks to come back. Julie interprets them and the results indicate that Maria has a dMMR tumour. The MMR immunohistochemistry test indicates a pathogenic variant in MSH2 – Maria's MSH2 proteins are absent. High MSI is identified, which suggests a diagnosis of LS, so it is indicated that germline testing should be offered. The test results and associated data have a record number for family members to give health care professionals to access the records.

Julie calculates the probability of being a carrier using clinical testing criteria to evaluate each member of the family. All of Maria's siblings, parents and children now know they have one first degree relative with confirmed LS-related cancer and another likely (Ann). Maria's sister Ann has a high probability of having LS because she has had endometrial cancer before age 50. Julie knows that it is important to think about the prevention of colorectal cancer in people with Lynch syndrome (NICE, 2021).

If Maria's parents both test, this could help to predict the risk of LS for their brothers and sisters and their children (Maria's aunts, uncles, and cousins). The results of the tumour test help Julie to order appropriate confirmatory germline tests for Maria's family members who consent to testing for the same variation of MSH2 and high MSI instability. Each individual is offered genetic counselling and provides informed consent, on separate forms, recording discussion about what information they wish to receive, following the test and what they are happy to share. All are given the option to opt out of receiving germline results.

The genetic counsellor informs Maria's children and her siblings' children about the reproductive risk of CMMR syndrome (this occurs when you get two mutations in the same MMR gene, one copy from each parent). Maria's children decide that if their results are positive for LS they will tell their children when they are older and can consent to testing if they wish.

Julie collaborates with the multi-disciplinary team and with Maria to plan Maria's care. The high MSI which contributed to a diagnosis of LS indicates that immunotherapy may be effective, and Maria chooses to be treated with monoclonal antibodies.

Blood cancers

Genomic information is rapidly becoming a more significant part of the management of haematological cancers. Similarly to other types of cancer, identification of specific mutations in the bone marrow and in blood can guide treatment decisions. Epigenetic changes which trigger mutations in some enzymes that affect gene expression have been identified in most cases of follicular lymphoma and a quarter of cases of acute myeloid leukaemia, which can support precision oncological treatment (Lesk, 2017). In acute myeloid leukaemia, conventional chemotherapy has low cure rates and is poorly tolerated, especially in older adults. Genetic and epigenetic targeted therapies in place of or used in addition to cytotoxic drugs can improve outcomes (Yang and Wang, 2018).

Genomics in paediatric oncology

Genomics can be of value within paediatric medicine where more rare tumours are observed. Healthcare for rare genetic conditions will improve over time as they are sequenced to collect information that guides research. Extracting clinically significant information from a cancer genome is valuable in paediatric diagnosis owing to the lack of exposure to carcinogens as an obvious cause for a childhood cancer. Genomic tests can help to pinpoint a variant quickly in children because in addition to inherited genetic alterations, adults may have multiple mutations from exposure to environmental factors throughout their lifetime, making it more difficult to determine a single or combined cause for a cancer.

Acute lymphoblastic leukaemia (ALL) is the most common paediatric cancer diagnosis. A child's risk of developing ALL is increased by a diagnosis of:

- Down syndrome;
- Fanconi anaemia, a rare inherited disorder of the blood cells;
- ataxia telangiectasia, a rare inherited neurological disorder; or
- Bloom syndrome, a rare inherited disorder which affects the skin (Cancer Research UK, 2021).

Congenital ALL, usually diagnosed within the first year of life is a much rarer but more aggressive form of ALL. In the UK, paediatric oncology services include 21 principal treatment centres and the turnaround time for genomic tests is 2–3 weeks. Information from tumour DNA can be extracted from the blood and used to select treatment by identifying targets for drug action such as specific cellular receptors. Although unlikely to replace conventional chemotherapy, which improves outcomes in 95% of cases of childhood leukaemia, precision oncology drugs may be used in combination with chemotherapy to further improve survival rates (Chang et al., 2013).

Principal treatment centres in the UK

- Royal Aberdeen Children's Hospital
- Edinburgh Royal Hospital for Sick Children
- Glasgow Royal Hospital for Sick Children
- Great North Children's Hospital, Newcastle
- Royal Belfast Hospital for Sick Children
- Our Lady's Children's Hospital, Crumlin
- Leeds General Infirmary
- Alder Hey Children's Hospital, Liverpool
- Sheffield Children's Hospital
- Royal Manchester Children's Hospital
- Nottingham Children's Hospital
- Leicester Children's Hospital
- Birmingham Children's Hospital
- John Radcliffe Children's Hospital, Oxford
- Cambridge University Hospital
- Bristol Royal Hospital for Children
- The Noah's Ark Children's Hospital for Wales, Cardiff
- Great Ormond Street Children's Hospital, London
- University College London Hospital
- Royal Marsden Hospital, London
- Southampton General Hospital

(Children's Cancer and Leukaemia Group, 2024.)

Monoclonal antibodies (such as rituximab) are synthetic immune proteins that attack cancer cells to cause cell death (Robinson et al., 2023). Blinatumomab is a monoclonal antibody which is reported to be 'kinder' than chemotherapy and has the benefit of being mobile (it can be delivered by a portable pump), which can improve a child's quality of life (BBC News, 2024).

Nurses can approach parents at the point of a child's diagnosis to discuss whole genome sequencing. The benefits of whole genome sequencing (WGS), which is becoming a more commonplace part of paediatric cancer care, include prognostic observations that can inform the clinical management of somatic or germline changes. The whole genome can also be examined for any variants that may affect future health

(Trotman et al., 2022). Information can be stored throughout the lifespan to inform future health care, but this raises ethical considerations about factors such as incidental findings or extraneous significant health information revealed by genomic tests, explored further in Chapter 6.

Nurses and cancer research

In addition to improved diagnosis and guidance on safe and effective treatment choices, other benefits of genomic data include the identification of individuals who may benefit from participating in research (Genomics England, 2023). Nurses often help patients to access appropriate studies, and many are offered the opportunity to be involved in a clinical trial to determine the effectiveness of a type of treatment or research exploring other areas of their patient journey (NICE, 2023). Information gained from trials not only informs treatment choices but also helps cancer nurses to manage side effects and improve quality of life for those receiving treatment (Macmillan Cancer Support, 2023B).

Cancer vaccines

The information in DNA is used to direct the synthesis of proteins when new body cells are created. Protein synthesis involves the copying of cell DNA into RNA within the cell nucleus (this is called transcription). Messenger RNA (mRNA) then leaves the cell nucleus and enters the cytoplasm to direct the synthesis of a protein through translation of this code by ribosomes, cellular organelles (Lesk, 2017). This is called the central dogma of molecular biology, and more information can be found about this process in Chapter 1.

Cancer vaccines are a type of immunotherapy. They are developed from a person's tumour DNA fragments in people who have cancer. Messenger RNA vaccines use the central dogma to identify individual genetic mutations and to help individuals' bodies to fight their cancer by activating their immune system. The targeted treatment finds and attacks cancer cells to prevent recurrence. The NHS Cancer Vaccine Launchpad is a project linking suitable NHS cancer patients with vaccine trials. The project aims to enable patients to participate as early as possible following diagnosis and contribute to the development of vaccines to fight cancer (UK Government, 2023A). Nursing staff in cancer vaccine trials are collecting data to inform vaccine development as part of the direct care team. This treatment has been used in the UK to treat melanoma but current research is focused on developing treatments for lung, kidney and bladder cancers (NHS England, 2023B).

> ### Learning activity
>
> - Access the following websites to read more about cancer vaccines:
>   - NHS cancer vaccine launch pad (https://www.england.nhs.uk/cancer/nhs-cancer-vaccine-launch-pad/);
>   - Personalised cancer vaccines (https://news.cancerresearchuk.org/2024/05/31/patients-to-access-trials-of-personalised-cancer-vaccines/);
>   - Lung cancer vaccine (https://www.uclh.nhs.uk/news/first-uk-patient-receives-innovative-lung-cancer-vaccine).

Oncology nursing specialist genomics skills

Patients are commonly diagnosed with a type of cancer that indicates that other family members should be tested for a genetic pre-disposition to this type of cancer. As genomic science develops, nurses will develop the skills to provide optimal care using new technologies to care for patients and for their relatives. Choosing the appropriate tests to identify all possible pathogenic variants which could be causing a person's cancer is essential to inform cascade testing within their family (Mahon, 2022). Core nursing skills are used to care for people from all genetic and lifestyle backgrounds and must be adaptable to each individual's journey (NICE, 2023).

🌳 Family health history

Many types of cancer are hereditary and because different types of cancer can be caused by the same familial variant, charting family histories in cancer care is a more detailed process than in other areas of practice. To inform genomic test selection linked to a cancer diagnosis, a family health history should include:

■ a three-generation pedigree (Mahon, 2016);
■ a review of patient and maternal and paternal medical history; and
■ identification of any previous germline tests, including tumour tests if available, and evaluation of results (Mahon, 2022; Holter et al., 2022; NICE, 2023).

Polygenic risk scores can also contribute to risk prediction among family members and identification of increased risk means that nurses must refer patients for appropriate screening or tests. When signposting patients to other services or professionals, nurses must provide appropriate counselling and ensure that they understand the potential implications of any actions and can give informed consent. There is a comprehensive process for obtaining consent for genomic tests during which patients will record their preferences in relation to receiving information and understanding the meaning of any possible results (Royal College of Physicians, London, 2019). The consent process is outlined more fully in Chapter 4 and confidentiality is explored in Chapter 6.

Specialist nurses must interpret and relay test results and support patients to make decisions based on these results. They possess skills in accessing the evidence base, finding relevant information and sharing this information with patients. A growing number of evidence-based guidelines can help with clinical decision making based on the application of the many new recommendations to practice (Puddester et al., 2022). Communication, as in all areas of nursing, must be comprehensive, clear and accurate. Oncology nurses assist patients to understand large amounts of complex information associated with genomic testing and the possible consequences of different treatment options (Friend, 2020). It is necessary that verbal or written information given by nurses is accessible, is given in the patient's preferred language and meets their individual literacy level (NICE, 2023). Nurses must also elicit individual values and preferences and religious or cultural needs (Jenkins, 2011). They are sometimes required to advocate for patients when managing treatment pathways that will take these needs into account (Allen, 2018).

Nurses provide emotional support and may signpost to other multidisciplinary services to meet holistic needs. Nurses who have a good awareness of available interventions can help people to cope with the impact of cancer treatments and surgeries; many cancer patients will experience altered body image and an impact on sexual function owing to factors such as pain, scarring, incontinence or stoma following surgery (NICE, 2021). Nurses can direct people to professionals who are well-placed to offer therapies to support well-being and reduce distress (Jeffers et al., 2019). Mental health can be affected by cancer journeys and part of the nursing role is also to provide individuals with the opportunity to highlight mental as well as physical signs and symptoms for review (Martin, 2020.)

🩺 Skills focus

Imagine you are a nurse preparing for a consultation. You will be seeing a young adult male with cancer who has previously reported altered body image and impaired sexual function.
   Think about (and perhaps research):

- what communication skills you might use to find out about and try to understand his experience and how he feels;
- what information you can share with him about managing his symptoms;
- other health care services he might wish to be referred to; and
- any other support services you can tell him about.

Supported recovery to improve health and quality of life for those who have cancer is a significant part of cancer nursing care. This includes, for example, giving information on diet, exercise and other lifestyle changes for cancer patients (University of Leicester, 2011). Cancer genome tests can help to predict the likelihood of breast cancer recurrence but when supporting patients, nurses must also take into account the 'social genome' or genes which can be affected by life experiences (Milani et al 2023, p.2). In addition to more commonly understood risk factors such as smoking and poor diet, epidemiological factors including social isolation and a sedentary lifestyle can increase the expression of pro-inflammatory genes and increase the likelihood of a cancer recurrence. Nurses can use this information to enhance risk assessment and work with patients in the context of their own lives and social resources to facilitate improved outcomes.

Self-awareness is a useful trait in nursing. When committing to the provision of person-centred care for others, it is important to recognise when one's own values may influence our practice. An awareness of the advantages of genomic testing might impact on information given to patients. It is important to remain as unbiased as possible, especially if there is a tension between what a nurse believes to be the best course of action and what a patient chooses (Jenkins, 2011). 'Enthusiasm' for tools such as polygenic risk scoring should not cloud judgment over when to use them or cause health care practitioners to overlook limitations (Sud et al., 2023, p.1).

Nurses are accountable for being competent in their roles. With the expansion of roles and new genomics tools, skills and knowledge, it can be difficult for individual specialist oncology nurses to define their scope of practice and to understand what knowledge and skills constitute competence. However, it is critical to remain up to date with developments in this field (Mahon, 2022) and competency frameworks or concept inventories can help to structure learning and development. These include:

- NHS England and Health Education England frameworks such as the genomic nursing proficiencies (NHS England, 2023A) and frameworks for those working in specialist areas such as the competency framework for genomic testing (Health Education England, 2021); and
- the genomic nursing concept inventory (Ward et al., 2014).

Nurse leadership in cancer care

The provision of quality care for individuals is central to nursing and nurses are instrumental within the bigger picture of precision oncology. As the largest group of health care practitioners, nurses are essential for the effective integration of genomics into health care. Genomics competent nurses have the knowledge, skills and experience to develop and improve services, including timely access to tests and treatment (Puddester et al., 2022).

Oncology nurses also have a role in educating the public. Understanding of social determinants of health can help them to empower communities to access screening and improve outcomes, particularly for those in minority ethnic and cultural groups (Allen, 2018). The support of organisations, the availability of effective education and the ability to attend educational opportunities is vital. This will support nurses to continue to take responsibility for ensuring that advances in genomics benefit all patients (Calzone et al., 2010). Nurse leaders acting effectively as role models increase the number of nurses within their organisations who consider genomics skills and knowledge to be an important part of a nurse's overall competency and oncology specialist nurses, in particular, clearly demonstrate how genomics can be integrated into care to improve outcomes (Calzone et al., 2018).

Ethical issues in cancer genomics

Individual or family situations surrounding genomic testing or receiving results can raise ethical questions which nurses must help patients to navigate and make balanced decisions on. Ethical decision making can be complex, and nurses often feel a burden of responsibility. Cancer diagnoses may lead to distressing treatment choices and carriers of pathogenic BRCA gene mutations may be offered preventive surgery for breast and ovarian cancer and the option to have breast tissue or ovaries and fallopian tubes removed. Nurses can use decision aids to help people to explore their options (NICE, 2023). Patients need enhanced support when making life-changing decisions and must be made aware of any potential psychological, psychosocial or psychosexual impact. It is imperative that health care practitioners can offer information and reassurance, but it may feel problematic to promote an intervention that may lead to harm, particularly when few effective strategies are available to maintain well-being (Jeffers et al., 2019).

> ### 📖 Learning activity – decision aids
>
> Patient decision aids incorporate information to support health professionals to help patients make a decision about the best tests or treatment for them. They are usually visual (for example a video, a chart, or a leaflet) and based on current evidence around available options.
>
> ■ Think about the utility of any patient decision aids you may have used in your practice.
> ■ Consider what a decision aid for types of cancer treatment might look like, to help a patient weigh up the advantages and limitations of the choices available to them.

Some decisions, for example those related to individual privacy and confidentiality, can have emotional implications for patients and families. Considering sharing genetic information and potentially significant test results with members of the family who are estranged, or those planning to have children, may feel overwhelming. The PiGeOn project is a recent Australian longitudinal study that aims to measure the psychosocial impact of germline genomic sequencing felt by families over time and to explore coping strategies (Best et al., 2018). This study will help to strengthen the process of informed consent for genomic testing. The results from this study may also enable nurses to reassure themselves that ethical considerations regarding potential patient distress, particularly when supporting those receiving uncertain results, are incorporated in practice.

> ### 📖 Learning activity – understanding patient experience
>
> Understanding an individual's experience of their genomics journey, including diagnosis, symptoms of disease, their treatment and its impact on their lives, is important in identifying needs and providing appropriate nursing care.
>
> ■ Search for a range of online resources which can help nurses to understand varied patient experiences of testing, diagnosis and treatment for cancer. You can mix and match search terms to access a range of results. A good example is healthtalk.org, a website where you can hear individuals' experiences of various health conditions including different cancers.
>
> (This learning activity is designed to support the achievement of NHS England (2023A) genomic nursing competency 8.)

Recording exactly which information a patient is happy to receive following a test becomes relevant when secondary findings present a familial disease risk not related to the condition tested for. Patient preferences may be influenced by individual or cultural values and failure to discuss preferences in advance can lead to an ethically and sometimes legally difficult situation for those receiving and for those reporting results (Hicks et al., 2021). Incidental findings from genomic tests are discussed further in Chapter 6.

Nurses may also face ethical issues related to equity of care in different regions. For those who pay for health care, genomic testing can be very expensive, especially testing for whole families, even when tests do not provide a definitive result. In the US, some financial aid and low-cost options are available for families who wish to have tests which are not covered by their health insurance. The Affordable Care Act means that insurance companies must pay for BRCA1 and BRCA 2 variant testing for women who meet specific criteria (Facing Our Risk.org, 2023). There is some variability in Medicaid programmes between states, but this legislation improves access to optimal care.

Nurses must also consider any potential harms that may result from care, including screening based on risk calculation. For example, if an increased risk of prostate cancer is identified and tests reveal the presence of a variant associated with cancer, patients may undergo invasive testing and experience distress without actually going on to develop prostate cancer. Increased risk scores do not change the existing process for prostate specific antigen testing and the screening process can unnecessarily affect quality of life for patients and their families (Sud et al., 2023).

Polygenic risk scores in cancer care

Polygenic risk scores (PRS) consider the combined effect of all identified variants within a person's genome to predict the risk of them developing a specific disease (Sud et al., 2023). The ability to calculate polygenic risk scores and to categorise levels of risk is expected to significantly advance health care (James et al., 2021).

The nursing role often includes holistic assessment and giving people information to protect their future health. Nurses routinely discuss the risks associated with smoking, excessive alcohol intake, unprotected exposure to the sun, processed foods and obesity. Lifestyle factors, health history and sometimes health care can exacerbate disease risks caused by genetic variation. For example, if a patient is suffering with menopausal symptoms and they have had oestrogen receptor positive breast or ovarian cancer, prescribing HRT can increase their risk of recurrence.

☼ Reflection point

- Imagine you are a 50-year-old woman recovering from oestrogen receptor positive breast cancer. You now have significant menopausal symptoms including hot flushes and vaginal dryness. You have been told that HRT is contraindicated for you.
- Think about the feelings you may have.
- Write down some ways in which a practice nurse might support your well-being.

An individual's risk of developing a disease can be estimated by using information from 500,000 participants on the association of common genetic variants with disease, collated by UK Biobank, a database of genetic information, explored further in Chapter 7. This information can be combined with patient factors such as age, sex and blood pressure to create an overall risk score. Risk factors are weighted according to the significance of their contribution to disease (HM Government, 2022).

BOADICEA (Breast and Ovarian Analysis of Disease Incidence and Carrier Estimation Algorithm) for predicting the risk of breast cancer incorporates the effects of common genetic variants and rare mutations in the known breast cancer susceptibility genes with family history, lifestyle and hormonal risk factors, and mammographic density (Lee et al., 2019). Use of this tool to calculate carrier probability is supported by NICE (2023) and scores can be used to guide screening schedules for individuals at risk.

Nurses must, however, have realistic expectations of what current risk scoring systems can offer and convey these expectations to patients. Practice should be consistent for polygenic risk scoring to be effective and PRS will be limited in disease prediction until there is one standardised tool that includes environmental factors and other non-genetic contributors in pathogenesis (Sud et al., 2023). Some patients fail to understand or engage with the data presented and this does not support the successful implementation of lifestyle changes to improve outcomes (Lewis et al., 2022).

Incidences of specific genetic variants vary between populations depending on ancestry. This means that risk scores will alter according to ethnic heritage. Building a bank of information on genetic markers for as many population groups as possible is important in improving accuracy for all individuals. Databases currently hold data from participants of mostly European descent and international efforts are focusing on ethnic diversity to improve PRS (HM Government, 2022). There are several populations globally for whom polygenic risk scoring is less informative, including people of African or Hispanic/Latin American ancestry, and nurses should take ancestry into account prior to discussing or calculating a polygenic risk score with a patient (James et al., 2021.)

Risk reduction

Health promotion for those at increased risk can have a greater positive impact than calculating a risk score (Sud et al., 2023). Raising awareness of common risks factors for cancer and disseminating information on how to lead a healthy lifestyle are central tenets of public health. Smoking cessation is mentioned above in relation to reducing the risk of developing lung cancer. Another example of where nurses make a difference can be seen in sexual and reproductive health. Nurses support the national cervical screening programme to increase uptake of routine cervical screening, particularly in areas where attendance is poor.

📖 **Learning activity – increasing uptake for cervical screening**

- Read this news article (https://www.gov.uk/government/news/new-national-cervical-screening-campaign-launches-as-nearly-1-in-3-dont-take-up-screening-offer) about increasing uptake for cervical cancer screening in the UK.
- Read this position statement (https://melanoma.org.au/wp-content/uploads/2024/02/MIA-Skin-Checks-for-Melanoma-Position-Statement.pdf) about melanoma detection and prevention in Australia.

Exposure to HPV through sexual contact increases the risk for cervical and throat cancers (Snyder, 2016). If a patient receives abnormal results from a smear test, this could be due to cellular changes (dysplasia) and may need further exploration.

Abnormal samples are tested for HPV. There are more than 200 types of HPV and 12 are considered to be high risk. Some strains (16 and 18) of HPV are oncogenic and can turn healthy cells into cancerous cells (National Cancer Institute, 2023). Some nursing roles include administration of the HPV vaccine, which causes the body to generate antibodies that stop HPV from spreading to other cells if a person is infected with the virus (UK Health Security Agency, 2023).

In addition to the provision of comprehensive care for individuals, many nurses raise awareness of the importance of testing for genetic variations which can increase cancer risk (Martin, 2020). Comprehensive knowledge helps nurses to take opportunities to give information when it is most needed to help people protect their health. People with lighter (less pigmented) skin are at increased risk of melanoma (Friend, 2020). It is reported that if genetic tests formed a bigger part of health promotion processes to encourage people to protect themselves from the harmful rays of the sun, particularly in hot countries such as Australia, then population outcomes would be improved. If people are aware that they are at increased risk of developing melanoma owing to the presence of a familial genetic variant, they may take greater care to protect their skin. Infrastructure should allow nurses to request these tests and to integrate this information into their practice (Primiero et al., 2022; Friend, 2020).

Whole genome sequencing and cancer

Genomic tests enable the detection of germline or inherited gene mutations, by examining specific parts of the genome for example, looking for changes in BRCA1 and BRCA2 genes. This helps health care professionals to evaluate an individual's risk of developing specific cancers as a result of these mutations, but unexplained incidences indicate that for some, other parts of the genome can affect outcomes.

Many people with BRCA1 mutations do not develop breast or ovarian cancer and this could be because a different part of the genome modifies the expression of this variant. On the other hand, some people with a mutation have no family history of breast or ovarian cancer, which means that the variation has arisen within their own genome (Lesk, 2017). Looking at *all* parts of the genome where variants can cause cancer can provide additional useful information.

In 2022, the UK Government announced a Cancer 2.0 programme led by Genomics England as a plan to realise a national genomics vision. This project will explore the use of WGS for cancers. Work to combine digital radiology and histopathology images with data from WGS will support research into improved diagnosis, prognosis and treatment response. Part of this plan involves using artificial intelligence to analyse genomic data (HM Government, 2022).

Skills and knowledge for all nurses

Lea et al. (2011) state that genomics is a rapidly changing field within which it is not expected that all nurses will have a comprehensive understanding. They conclude, however, that an awareness of how genomics can significantly benefit patient care and the ability to refer to identify need and refer to appropriate professionals are integral to effective nursing care. In addition to a family history, recognising other red flags for inherited cancers is important and useful in all areas of care.

⚑ Red flags for an inherited cancer

This knowledge is crucial to early diagnosis for patients and good outcomes in families and includes indicators such as:

- unusually severe presentation;
- bilateral presentation in paired organs;
- presentation of a patient who is below the typical age range associated with the condition;
- an absence of associated environmental factors; and
- a patient of a biological sex in which the condition less commonly occurs (e.g. breast cancer in men) (Primary Care Genetics, 2017).

Summary

The UK health care system is adapting to support the integration of genomic informed health care.

Identification and action to decrease the risk of disease forms part of all nursing roles and all nurses have a responsibility to meet professional body proficiencies, including genetics and genomics related care (Calzone et al., 2010). There are two levels of genomics competence in nursing and basic competence is required by all nurses regardless of specialty (Chair et al., 2019). This chapter has explored some core nursing skills alongside advanced skills for oncology nurses, including specialist knowledge and effective communication.

Learn more

- A free educational resource for primary care health care practitioners and students can be found at the Jackson Laboratory website. The Jackson Laboratory is an independent, non-profit biomedical research institution in Maine, USA: https://education.clinical.jax.org/page/hereditarycancerprogram
- The Oncology Nursing Society offers a free online course in how molecular biomarkers guide cancer treatment: https://www.ons.org/learning-libraries/precision-oncology
- Gateway C offers a free, accredited course for primary care staff in the identification of sarcoma: https://www.gatewayc.org.uk/courses/sarcoma/

Resources for patients

- The Centre for Genetics Education in New South Wales, Australia, has designed a free, comprehensive cancer genetics fact sheet: https://www.genetics.edu.au/PDF/Cancer_genetics_fact_sheet-CGE.pdf
- Another useful source of information is a series of short podcasts and YouTube videos produced by the University of Leicester (2011). This resource is for patients and includes information about cancer symptoms, genetic testing and inheritance patterns: https://le.ac.uk/vgec/topics/gene-mutations-and-cancer

- Macmillan Cancer Support provide detailed, accessible information on their website about different types of clinical trials in which patients who have cancer might be offered the opportunity to participate: https://www.macmillan.org.uk/cancer-information-and-support/treatments-and-drugs/clinical-trials
- Prostate cancer UK provides a range of useful information for patients with prostate cancer and the opportunity to ask their specialist nurses questions: https://prostatecanceruk.org/prostate-information-and-support

References

Allen, D., 2018. Genetic Testing: How genetics and genomics can affect healthcare disparities. *Clinical Journal of Oncology Nursing*, 22(1).

Allen, D., 2021. Cancer nursing and genomics. *Cancer Nursing Practice*, 20(2), 17–19. https://doi.org/10.7748/cnp.20.2.17.s10

BBC News, 2024. Exciting new cancer drug kinder than chemotherapy – BBC News. bbc.co.uk/news/health-67793887 (accessed 17 January 2024).

Best, M., Newson, A.J., Meiser, B., Juraskova, I., Goldstein, D., Tucker, K., Ballinger, M.L., Hess, D., Schlub, T.E., Biesecker, B. and Vines, R., 2018. The PiGeOn project: protocol of a longitudinal study examining psychosocial and ethical issues and outcomes in germline genomic sequencing for cancer. *BMC Cancer*, 18(1), pp.1–10.

Buaki-Sogo, M. and Percival, N., 2022. Genomic medicine: the role of the nursing workforce. *Nurs. Times*, 118, pp.1–3.

Calzone, K.A., Cashion, A., Feetham, S., Jenkins, J., Prows, C.A., Williams, J.K. and Wung, S.F., 2010. Nurses transforming health care using genetics and genomics. *Nursing Outlook*, 58(1), pp.26–35.

Calzone, K.A., Jenkins, J., Culp, S. and Badzek, L., 2018. Hospital nursing leadership-led interventions increased genomic awareness and educational intent in Magnet settings. *Nursing Outlook*, 66(3), pp.244–253.

Cancer Research UK, 2021. ALL. https://www.cancerresearchuk.org/about-cancer/acute-lymphoblastic-leukaemia-all/risks-causes (accessed 20 February 2024).

Cancer Research UK, 2023. Genes, DNA and cancer. https://www.cancerresearchuk.org/about-cancer/what-is-cancer/genes-dna-and-cancer (accessed 12 October 2023).

Chair, S.Y., Waye, M.M.Y., Calzone, K. and Chan, C.W.H., 2019. Genomics education in nursing in Hong Kong, Taiwan and mainland China. *International Nursing Review*, 66(4), pp.459–466.

Chan, R.J., Teleni, L., McDonald, S., Kelly, J., Mahony, J., Ernst, K., Patford, K., Townsend, J., Singh, M. and Yates, P., 2020. Breast cancer nursing interventions and clinical effectiveness: a systematic review. *BMJ Supportive & Palliative Care*, 10(3), pp.276–286.

Chang, V.Y., Basso, G., Sakamoto, K.M. and Nelson, S.F., 2013. Identification of somatic and germline mutations using whole exome sequencing of congenital acute lymphoblastic leukaemia. *BMC Cancer*, 13(1), pp.1–6.

Chatterjee, N. and Walker, G.C., 2017. Mechanisms of DNA damage, repair, and mutagenesis. *Environmental and Molecular Mutagenesis*, 58(5), pp.235–263.

Chen, Y., Williams, V., Filippova, M., Filippov, V. and Duerksen-Hughes, P., 2014. Viral carcinogenesis: factors inducing DNA damage and virus integration. *Cancers*, 6(4), pp.2155–2186.

Children's Cancer and Leukaemia Group, 2024. Specialist hospitals https://www.cclg.org.uk/In-hospital/Specialist-hospitals (accessed 25 October 2024).

Chung, C., 2022. Predictive and prognostic biomarkers with therapeutic targets in colorectal cancer: a 2021 update on current development, evidence, and recommendation. *Journal of Oncology Pharmacy Practice*, 28(4), pp.850–869.

Esposito, A., Criscitiello, C., Trapani, D. and Curigliano, G., 2017. The emerging role of 'liquid biopsies,' circulating tumor cells, and circulating cell-free tumor dna in lung cancer diagnosis and identification of resistance mutations. *Current Oncology Reports, 19*, pp.1–6.

Facing Our Risk.org, 2013. Insurance and paying for care. https://www.facingourrisk. org/support/insurance-paying-for-care/paying-for-genetic-services (accessed 14 November 2023).

Fee-Schroeder, K. and King, E., 2019. What is the difference between genetics and genomics? https://voice.ons.org/news-and-views/what-is-the-difference-between-genetics-and-genomics?ref=CO&&pk_vid=bda837a04bf3fd83168967167419fd84 (accessed 19 February 2024).

Friend, P., 2020. Biomarkers in cutaneous melanoma: implications for patient education and support. *Clinical Journal of Oncology Nursing, 24*(6), pp.660–666.

Genomics England, 2023. Cancer genomics. https://www.genomicsengland.co.uk/genomic-medicine/understanding-genomics/cancer-genomics (accessed 7 November 2023).

Gutierrez, C. and Schiff, R., 2011. HER2: biology, detection, and clinical implications. *Archives of Pathology & Laboratory Medicine, 135*(1), pp.55–62.

Health Education England, 2019. Cancer and the genome. https://www.genomicseducation.hee. nhs.uk/documents/cancer-and-the-genome/ (accessed 10 October 2023).

Health Education England, 2021. Facilitating genomic testing: a competency framework. https:// www.genomicseducation.hee.nhs.uk/competency-frameworks/consent-a-competency-framework/ (accessed 29 May 2025).

Hicks, J.K., Howard, R., Reisman, P., Adashek, J.J., Fields, K.K., Gray, J.E., McIver, B., McKee, K., O'Leary, M.F., Perkins, R.M. and Robinson, E., 2021. Integrating somatic and germline next-generation sequencing into routine clinical oncology practice. *JCO Precision Oncology, 5*, pp.884–895.

HM Government, 2022. Genome UK: 2022 to 2025 implementation plan for England. https:// www.gov.uk/government/publications/genome-uk-2022-to-2025-implementation-plan-for-england/genome-uk-2022-to-2025-implementation-plan-for-england

Holter, S., Hall, M.J., Hampel, H., Jasperson, K., Kupfer, S.S., Larsen Haidle, J., Mork, M.E., Palaniapppan, S., Senter, L., Stoffel, E.M. and Weissman, S.M., 2022. Risk assessment and genetic counseling for Lynch syndrome – practice resource of the National Society of Genetic Counselors and the Collaborative Group of the Americas on Inherited Gastrointestinal Cancer. *Journal of Genetic Counseling, 31*(3), pp.568–583.

James, J.E., Riddle, L., Koenig, B.A. and Joseph, G., 2021. The limits of personalization in precision medicine: Polygenic risk scores and racial categorization in a precision breast cancer screening trial. *PLoS One, 16*(10), p.e0258571.

Jasperson, K.W., Tuohy, T.M., Neklason, D.W. and Burt, R.W., 2010. Hereditary and familial colon cancer. *Gastroenterology, 138*(6), pp.2044–2058.

Jeffers, L., Reid, J., Fitzsimons, D., Morrison, P.J. and Dempster, M., 2019. Interventions to improve psychosocial well-being in female BRCA-mutation carriers following risk-reducing surgery. *Cochrane Database of Systematic Reviews, 10.* https://doi.org/10.1002/14651858. CD012894.pub2

Jenkins, J., 2011, February. Essential genetic and genomic nursing competencies for the oncology nurse. *Seminars in Oncology Nursing, 27*(1), pp.64–71).

Lea, D.H., Skirton, H., Read, C.Y. and Williams, J.K., 2011. Implications for educating the next generation of nurses on genetics and genomics in the 21st century. *Journal of Nursing Scholarship, 43*(1), pp.3–12.

Lee, A., Mavaddat, N., Wilcox, A.N., Cunningham, A.P., Carver, T., Hartley, S., Babb de Villiers, C., Izquierdo, A., Simard, J., Schmidt, M.K. and Walter, F.M., 2019. BOADICEA: a comprehensive breast cancer risk prediction model incorporating genetic and nongenetic risk factors. *Genetics in Medicine, 21*(8), pp.1708–1718.

Lesk, A.M., 2017. *Introduction to Genomics.* Oxford University Press, Oxford.

Lewis, A.C., Perez, E.F., Prince, A.E., Flaxman, H.R., Gomez, L., Brockman, D.G., Chandler, P.D., Kerman, B.J., Lebo, M.S., Smoller, J.W. and Weiss, S.T., 2022. Patient and provider perspectives on polygenic risk scores: implications for clinical reporting and utilization. *Genome Medicine*, 14(1), p.114.

Macmillan Cancer Support, 2022. Inherited bowel cancer. https://www.macmillan.org.uk/cancer-information-and-support/worried-about-cancer/causes-and-risk-factors/inherited-bowel-cancer (accessed 7 January 2024).

Macmillan Cancer Support, 2023A. Family history, genes and cancer risk. https://www.macmillan.org.uk/cancer-information-and-support/worried-about-cancer/causes-and-risk-factors/family-history-genetics-and-cancer-risk (accessed 14 November 2023).

Macmillan Cancer Support, 2023B. Clinical trials https://www.macmillan.org.uk/cancer-information-and-support/treatments-and-drugs/clinical-trials (accessed 9 November 2023).

Mahon, S.M., 2016. The three-generation pedigree: a critical tool in cancer genetics care. *Oncology Nursing Forum*, 43(5), pp.655–660.

Mahon, S.M., 2022. Oncology nurse practitioners in genetics: examining scope of practice and competence. *Clinical Journal of Oncology Nursing*, 26(2), pp.141–145.

Martin, J.C., 2020. Genetic biomarkers: implications of increased understanding and identification in lung cancer management. *Clinical Journal of Oncology Nursing*, 24(6), pp.648–656.

MHRA, 2024. Biobank. Yellow Card biobank | Making medicines and medical devices safer. https://yellowcard.mhra.gov.uk/biobank (accessed 19 February 2024).

Milani, A., Misurelli, E., Bottaccioli, A.G., Bottaccioli, F., Lacapra, S., Ciccarelli, C., Magon, G. and Mazzocco, K., 2023. The iceberg of genomics: new perspectives in the use of genomics and epigenetics in oncology nursing clinical reasoning. A discursive paper. *Journal of Advanced Nursing*, 79(12), pp.4560–4567. https://doi.org/10.1111/jan.15858

Moore, L. and Hayes, A.E., 2023. Cancer health literacy in black women with breast cancer: a comprehensive literature review. *Clinical Journal of Oncology Nursing*, 27(5), pp.507–513.

National Cancer Institute, 2023. HPV and cancer. https://www.cancer.gov/about-cancer/causes-prevention/risk/infectious-agents/hpv-and-cancer (accessed 4 November 2023).

NHS, 2022. Live well quit smoking. https://www.nhs.uk/live-well/quit-smoking/nhs-stop-smoking-services-help-you-quit/ (accessed 19 February 2024).

NHS England, 2022. National Genomic Test Directory. https://www.england.nhs.uk/publication/national-genomic-test-directories/ (accessed 25 January 2024).

NHS England, 2023A. The 2023 Genomic Competency Framework for UK Nurses. https://www.genomicseducation.hee.nhs.uk/wp-content/uploads/2023/12/2023-Genomic-Competency-Framework-for-UK-Nurses.pdf (accessed 29 May 2025).

NHS England, 2023B. Cancer vaccine launchpad. https://www.england.nhs.uk/contact-us/privacy-notice/how-we-use-your-information/public-and-partners/cancer-vaccine-launchpad/ (accessed 16 December 2023).

NHS England, 2024. News. https://www.england.nhs.uk/2024/02/nhs-launches-national-brca-gene-testing-programme-to-identify-cancer-risk-early/ (accessed 19 February 2024).

NICE, 2017. DG27 Molecular testing strategies for Lynch syndrome in people with colorectal cancer. Overview. https://www.nice.org.uk/guidance/dg27 (accessed 20 February 2024).

NICE, 2021. NG151. Colorectal cancer. Overview. https://www.nice.org.uk/guidance/ng151 (accessed 20 February 2024).

NICE, 2023. CG164. https://www.nice.org.uk/guidance/cg164/chapter/Recommendations#clinical-significance-of-a-family-history-of-breast-cancer (accessed 19 February 2024).

North Thames GMS, 2024. News. https://norththamesgenomics.nhs.uk/circulating-tumour-testing-in-the-nhs/

Pettitt, S.J. and Lord, C.J., 2019. Dissecting PARP inhibitor resistance with functional genomics. *Current Opinion in Genetics & Development*, 54, pp.55–63.

Primary Care Genetics, 2017. Red flags for clinical practice. https://www.primarycaregenetics.org/ (accessed 24 November 2023).

Primiero, C.A., Baker, A.M., Wallingford, C.K., Maas, E.J., Yanes, T., Fowles, L., Janda, M., Young, M.A., Nisselle, A., Terrill, B. and Lodge, J.M., 2022. Attitudes of Australian dermatologists on the use of genetic testing: A cross-sectional survey with a focus on melanoma. *Frontiers in Genetics*, 13, p.3062.

Puddester, R., Pike, A., Maddigan, J. and Farrell, A., 2022. Nurses' knowledge, attitudes, confidence, and practices with genetics and genomics: a theory-informed integrative review protocol. *Journal of Personalized Medicine*, 12(9), p.1358.

Read, C.Y. and Ward, L.D., 2018. Misconceptions about genomics among nursing faculty and students. *Nurse Educator*, 43(4), pp.196–200.

Robinson, S.L., Seneviratne, N. and Dandapani, M., 2023. Understanding recent advances in genomic testing in paediatric oncology. *Paediatrics and Child Health*, 34(2), pp.43–48.

Royal College of Physicians. London 2019. Consent and confidentiality in genomic medicine. Consent and confidentiality in genomic medicine. https://www.rcplondon.ac.uk/projects/outputs/consent-and-confidentiality-genomic-medicine (accessed 19 February 2024).

Snyder, M., 2016. *Genomics and Personalized Medicine: What Everyone Needs to Know*. Oxford University Press.

Specialist Pharmacy Service, 2022. Medication restrictions for patients having CAR T-cell therapy. https://www.sps.nhs.uk/articles/medication-restrictions-for-patients-having-car-t-cell-therapy/ (accessed 21 February 2024).

St Mark's Hospital, 2019. *Lynch Syndrome: Information for Patients*. North West Thames Regional Genetics Service.

Sud, A., Horton, R.H., Hingorani, A.D., Tzoulaki, I., Turnbull, C., Houlston, R.S. and Lucassen, A., 2023. Realistic expectations are key to realising the benefits of polygenic scores. *bmj*, 380, https://doi.org/10.1136/bmj-2022-073149

Trotman, J., Armstrong, R., Firth, H., Trayers, C., Watkins, J., Allinson, K., Jacques, T.S., Nicholson, J.C., Burke, G.A. and Behjati, S., 2022. The NHS England 100,000 Genomes Project: feasibility and utility of centralised genome sequencing for children with cancer. *British Journal of Cancer*, 127(1), pp.137–144.

UK Government, 2023A. Press release. https://www.gov.uk/government/news/major-agreement-to-deliver-new-cancer-vaccine-trials (accessed 23 October 2023)

UK Government, 2023B. Press release. https://www.gov.uk/government/news/mhra-authorises-enzyme-inhibitor-anastrozole-to-prevent-breast-cancer-in-post-menopausal-women. (accessed 7 November 2023)

UK Health Security Agency, 2023. HPV vaccination guidance for healthcare practitioners. https://www.gov.uk/government/publications/hpv-universal-vaccination-guidance-for-health-professionals/hpv-vaccination-guidance-for-healthcare-practitioners (accessed 19 February 2024).

University of Leicester, 2011. Diet for cancer patients. https://le.ac.uk/vgec/topics/gene-mutations-and-cancer (accessed 19 February 2023).

Vu, T. and Claret, F.X., 2012. Trastuzumab: updated mechanisms of action and resistance in breast cancer. *Frontiers in Oncology*, 2, p.62.

Ward, Linda D., Mel Haberman, and Celestina Barbosa-Leiker, 2014. Development and psychometric evaluation of the genomic nursing concept inventory. *Journal of Nursing Education*, 53(9), pp.511–518.

Yang, X. and Wang, J., 2018. Precision therapy for acute myeloid leukemia. *Journal of Hematology & Oncology*, 11(1), pp.1–11.

Young, A.M., Charalambous, A., Owen, R.I., Njodzeka, B., Oldenmenger, W.H., Alqudimat, M.R. and So, W.K., 2020. Essential oncology nursing care along the cancer continuum. *The Lancet Oncology*, 21(12), pp.e555–e563.

CHAPTER 6

Genomics, ethics and the law

Chapter outline

This chapter explores some of the ethical and legal challenges associated with genomic medicine and sources of support for nurses navigating these issues in practice. Common issues include protecting privacy and confidentiality when sharing genomic data, inequality of service provision and ethical questions linked to gene therapy.

Introduction

The benefits of genomic medicine and whole genome sequencing include diagnostic and prognostic efficiency and accuracy and the development and use of targeted treatment to improve outcomes for patients. They also include surveillance and cascade testing for families, which could result in early diagnosis of genetic conditions or preventative measures. Genomic test results can inform reproductive decisions and pharmacogenetic data can improve medicines safety. However, in addition to the many benefits there are some significant risks, and it is important that people understand the implications of all possible test results for themselves and their families. Testing can raise challenges for patients precipitating difficult conversations. Feelings of guilt or feelings of blame towards others can affect relationships and family dynamics, leaving people in need of support.

Following the Human Genome Project, increased knowledge about gene function has led to a number of ethical, legal and social concerns. These concerns must be addressed by researchers and health services, but most importantly, by nurses (Nicol, 2002). Nurses can help patients to address ethical questions, and comprehensive guidance from the organisations within which they work will ensures nurses can practise within the law and avoid some common challenges, for example, processes related to consent, sharing information, testing other members of the family or health insurance.

DOI: 10.4324/9781003453048-6

Informed consent

Informed consent to test cannot be provided until accurate information has been given effectively by nurses and understood by patients. Information about the potential implications of testing should be raised for all patients offered a genetic test because, while the public have general familiarity with some genetic and health terminology, there may be some gaps. Information can be given in various formats prior to discussion with a health care practitioner to allow patients to prepare. Services should be equipped with written and visual materials at different levels of literacy and in languages appropriate to the local community. Supporting written information can be given to patients during consultations to review at home (Strategic Reform and Planning, 2021).

Many patient questions focus on practical aspects of testing, receiving results and completing associated documentation (Sanderson et al., 2019). There should be written information available for patients about the organisation's policy for keeping personal information safe (Strategic Reform and Planning, 2021). Health providers must also have local protocols to guide nurses obtaining consent for genomic tests to ensure that each patient is given all of the information they need about the processes involved and what each aspect for which they are providing consent means for them (Strategic Reform and Planning, 2021). In addition to these details, when giving consent to test patients should receive information about how their genomic data can have implications for family members. They should be prompted to consider any potentially difficult situations, and this discussion should be documented and retained as a record of topics covered (Tluczek et al., 2019).

Records should outline patient preferences for receiving genomic information supplementary to the test requested. For example, if a family is testing for pathological BRCA variants as the cause of a suspected heritable cancer but other conditions (for example Parkinson's disease) have appeared within the family, it should be clearly stated which information is to be given from any potential results. Screening the whole genome, when multiple gene panels are examined for variants, increases the likelihood of incidental findings; if a person has a suspected cardiac condition a whole cardiac panel might be requested, including tests for the suspected variant and for other related conditions.

Nurses can support people to make decisions about the tests they want by sharing current evidence and using decision aids. These resources should be utilised prior to the consent process for any intervention so patients are not receiving information that may affect their decision making at the time they are expected to sign the consent form. Individuals should be given time to consider their options and the opportunity to ask questions.

Nurses must be confident to raise issues for consideration with patients and to make clear all potential outcomes. They must be accomplished communicators with the ability to show empathy for everyone in their care. Individualised information about genomic tests helps patients to feel supported and to prepare for a range of outcomes. The consent process will often incorporate a discussion around balancing potential benefits with potential negative considerations (Sanderson et al., 2019). The Genomics Education Programme contains a competency framework to guide the genomic testing and consent process. This framework (Health Education England, 2021) helps nurses to be systematic and to practise according to UK law.

Genomic testing competencies

1. Ensures the process of recording consent for a genomic test follows national and local processes and governance arrangements, and is appropriate for the test being requested.
2. Demonstrates up-to-date knowledge of the conditions occurring within their specialist area for which genetic or genomic testing may be offered.
3. Assesses where genomic testing is appropriate in the patient's clinical pathway.
4. Conveys to patients the purpose and process of the clinical test being offered.
5. Explains and answers questions relating to the National Genomic Research Library where applicable.
6. Applies core clinical skills to the genomic test conversation.
7. Recognises one's ongoing responsibilities to the patient and acts when appropriate.
8. Seeks further assistance, where relevant, based on scope of practice.

(Health Education England, 2021.)

Many potential issues for consideration and discussion with patients prior to testing, including implications for patients, their families and wider implications appear on the NHS England (2021) Genomic Medicine Service Record of Discussion form, which is a tool designed to help ensure that all important aspects of testing are discussed. This record forms part of the consent form and a separate Record of Discussion form must be completed for each patient applying for a genomic test and on behalf of each child for whom parents are providing consent.

 Skills focus

■ Write your own checklist of topics to discuss in order to ensure informed consent to a genomic test.
■ Compare your checklist to the NHS England (2021) record of discussion form (https://www.england.nhs.uk/wp-content/uploads/2021/09/nhs-genomic-medicine-service-record-of-discussion-form.pdf) and note any differences.

Capacity to consent

Nurses are often required to assess a person's ability to understand and recall information and in this way they can ensure that all patients are equipped to manage different aspects of their care. Patients have varying levels of literacy and cognitive abilities. Nurses must not assume that all patients have the same basic knowledge and must ascertain the amount and level of information required for each individual, which will enable them to provide informed consent. In addition to the effective provision of information, health care professionals obtaining consent for genomic tests must also have the skills to elicit information about patients' views, to listen in order to understand concerns and be equipped to answer a range of questions (Sanderson et al., 2019).

If a nurse thinks it would benefit them, but a patient declines to access testing, capacity must be assumed. People have the right to make choices that are not aligned with advice and recommendations given by health care practitioners (Joint Committee on Genomics in Medicine, 2019). However, some patients who may benefit from genomic testing or treatment for a genetic variant or risk may have a learning disability or another condition affecting their capacity to give consent. Many such patients will have somebody who advocates for them and can make decisions on their behalf. Healthcare practitioners can make 'best interest' decisions if assessment shows that a person lacks the capacity to consent to tests or treatment. In these cases, Deprivation of Liberty Safeguards should be in place for use by the multidisciplinary team. Any interventions made must represent the least restrictive option for the individual's rights and freedoms (Mental Capacity Act, UK Government, 2005).

Ethical challenges may be raised on behalf of adults who lack the capacity to consent to a genetic test if the results will not be of immediate benefit to them but will inform the diagnosis or treatment of a member of their family, for example tests for a suspected BRCA variant or for Lynch syndrome (Joint Committee on Genomics in Medicine, 2019). In this situation, nurses can act as advocates for patients and need to understand the clinical value of any proposed test and if results will precipitate diagnosis, treatment or improved quality of life. Nurses may have to negotiate within challenging family dynamics to safeguard a patient.

Consenting to genetic tests for children

Parents or legal guardians are often required to make health-related decisions on behalf of children. Under 16s are presumed not to have the capacity to consent to genomic tests and if a test result will inform their immediate care, it is appropriate to make a best interest decision for them.

In some circumstances best interests can be a subjective position, and genomic tests may raise ethical questions about revealing certain information. It may be that an individual would strongly prefer not to know about an inherited pre-disposition to a future disease. Nurses may have to use ethical principles to balance the ability to predict the development of degenerative conditions and the potential impact on the lifestyle and mental health. In such cases testing should be offered only if preventive or delaying treatment is available and early diagnosis is beneficial (Joint Committee on Genomics in Medicine, 2019).

Genetic tests might be a precursor to invasive treatment such as gene therapy or distressing experiences for a child and some diagnoses can lead to stigmatisation and discrimination throughout their lifetime (*ABC v. St George's Healthcare NHS Trust*, 2015). Some under 16s may be assessed as Gillick competent to make their own decisions about such tests and treatments if they are provided with adequate information and support (Joint Committee on Genomics in Medicine, 2019). The American Society for Human Genetics, however, recognises the potential psychological impact of the identification of increased risk for children and adolescents. They recommend that adolescents are encouraged to defer testing for adult-onset conditions to avoid receiving significant information during 'formative' years (*ABC v. St George's Healthcare NHS Trust*, 2015, p.8). In addition to psychosocial considerations, relevant ethical factors should be explored. Unless testing would lead to an appropriate clinical intervention in childhood, delaying testing until adulthood supports a child's freedom (*ABC v. St George's Healthcare NHS Trust*, 2015).

As with adults who lack capacity, tests for which the results will benefit others but not the child themselves are also ethically challenging to manage.

🔍 Case study

This fictional case study was adapted from a case study (Case 6: Testing children for future-relevant information) within the Royal College of Physicians guidance (Joint Committee on Genomics in Medicine, 2019).

A baby, Anneka, who was tested for cystic fibrosis via the newborn screening programme, was found to be a carrier of a genetic variant for cystic fibrosis. Based on this information, her parents requested carrier testing for their older daughter Pippi, aged 6. Knowing Pippi's carrier status will not affect her medical care but may be of importance to her when she reaches reproductive age. If she is a carrier and her future partner is a carrier of the same variant, there will be a 2 in 4 chance of each of their children being born with cystic fibrosis.

Key points:

- The purpose of the newborn screening programme is to identify babies with genetic conditions so that they can have early treatment, aiming to improve prognosis, not to identify babies who are carriers of conditions. Discovery of carrier status is an incidental finding in a small proportion of families.
- Testing Pippi for cystic fibrosis carrier status has no medical benefit for the child, and current professional guidance is that testing should be deferred until she is old enough to make her own decision.
- Testing children for genetic variants that will only be of relevance to them once they are adults is usually considered beyond the boundaries of parental consent.

Data storage

Nurses must be competent to record, manage and securely store genetic and other health data. They have a responsibility to restrict access to this information in order to practice legally (Tluczek et al., 2019). General Data Protection Regulation requires that patients understand that there is strong legal protection for health information and that it should be made clear what their information will be used for (Data Protection Act, UK Government, 2018B).

Employer organisations can help nurses by having clear, service level guidelines for safeguarding data and the necessary sharing of genetic information.

⚖️ Caldicott Principles

The eight Caldicott Principles are national guidelines to support health organisations to ensure proper treatment of patient-identifying information:

- justify the purpose(s) for using confidential information;
- use confidential information only when it is necessary;

- use the minimum necessary confidential information;
- access to confidential information should be on a strict need-to-know basis;
- everyone with access to confidential information should be aware of their responsibilities;
- comply with the law;
- the duty to share information for individual care is as important as the duty to protect patient confidentiality; and
- inform patients and service users about how their confidential information is used (National Data Guardian, 2020).

Storage and access to genomic data should be discussed in advance of any genetic test and when obtaining consent for whole genome screening, and this skill forms part of the nursing competency framework for facilitating genomic testing (Health Education England, 2021). Patients in the UK can choose to have their data entered into the National Genomic Research Library. This information can be accessed to inform future health decisions within their life. Healthcare practitioners involved in their care will also have access to this data. National and international health researchers must apply to see the data. Insurance companies and other national organisations cannot access it. Patients who give consent and change their minds can have their data removed from the library.

DNA storage

The Human Tissue Act (UK Government, 2004) requires appropriate consent for all health-related tests, storage and research using samples from live subjects. Patients must sign the NHS (2021) Genomics Medicine Service record of discussion form which includes the statement that:

> Normal NHS laboratory practice is to store the DNA extracted from my sample even after my current testing is complete. My DNA might be used for future analysis and/or to ensure that other testing (for example that of family members) is of high quality.

DNA samples are routinely stored and may be used again as quality assurance for the testing process. It is sometimes necessary to look at past test results to develop interpretation processes and total anonymity cannot always be guaranteed in these circumstances as things like gender or ethnicity might be an important factor (Joint Committee on Genomics in Medicine, 2019). It is also possible that retained samples may be used for secondary research purposes to advance scientific discovery and consent for the future use of samples should be attained separately to any consent given for current clinical use (Strategic Reform and Planning, 2021).

Sharing results within families

A common example of an ethically problematic situation is when genetic test results have implications for family members, but patients do not wish to share their genetic information. Nurses may feel an obligation to disclose information that may affect the future health of relatives but be unsure about the ethics underpinning potential courses of action. A nurse's primary duty of care, including respect for their confidentiality, is to their patient (Tluczek et al., 2019). Nurses may sometimes be unsure about when information about an inherited genetic risk or variant can be communicated to family members.

Test results might initiate cascade testing and early intervention, improving outcome for others. Balancing a patient's privacy with the duty of care to relatives can be challenging and nurses must carefully balance these rights (Joint Committee on Genomics in Medicine, 2019). Healthcare professionals may be able to avoid breaching the confidentiality of an individual by disclosing information relating only to the family health status (Dove et al., 2019). Research increasingly supports a 'relational' approach of genomic tests and data to enable health care practitioners to care effectively for families (Weller et al., 2022).

The General Medical Council permits doctors to disclose health information if they can prevent harm by doing so (Dove et al., 2019). General Data Protection Regulation does not obstruct good care and respect for the privacy of patients should not prevent health professionals from advising other related individuals about identified risks to their health (Joint Committee on Genomics in Medicine, 2019).

Dove et al. (2019) highlight the case of *ABC v. St George's Healthcare NHS Trust and others*, which was brought against health care practitioners who did not disclose to a woman, in line with her father's wishes not to, that her father had been diagnosed with Huntington's disease. The woman, who was pregnant, felt that she may have decided not to continue with the pregnancy had she known that she may go on to develop the disease. In the absence of precedent, the court of appeal decided in 2017 that it was possible to recognise a duty of care to genetic relatives within the law if a benefit could be demonstrated to support the disclosure of information relevant to their health.

Patients having a single genetic test can keep their information private but people accessing whole genome sequencing (WGS) must consent to information discovered that affects other members of their family being shared with them.

🔍 Case study – privacy and confidentiality

This fictional case study outlines an example of common difficulties faced by patients, families, and genomics nurses.

Orla is 55 and has breast cancer. She has been offered a genetic test by the oncology specialist nurse and doesn't want to have it. Orla has a daughter, Kay, who wants her mum to take the test to find out whether the cancer was caused by an inherited genetic variation. Kay has a son and a daughter both aged under 5. Kay knows that if her mum tests, this will improve the predictive accuracy of any test she has. Kay wants to know whether she, and her daughter, will be at increased risk of developing breast cancer in the future. She has also heard that boys can get breast cancer too.

Orla's grandmother died following extensive 'women's trouble' and Kay suspects that this was a euphemism for a gynaecological cancer. She worries that it was ovarian cancer because she thinks she has read that having a BRCA gene variation can cause both breast cancer and ovarian cancer.

Orla is currently undergoing treatment with chemotherapy and feels like she has been through enough. She is distressed at the thought of knowing there is something genetically wrong with her and even more distressed that she might have unknowingly passed on a faulty gene.

Kay is increasingly frustrated and, when at the hospital, asks the oncology nurse for advice.

What could the nurse do?

■ Offer to record a family health history for Kay and discuss her individual risk.

■ Ask Orla and Kay if they want to talk together. Respect Orla's right to refuse and her confidentiality if she declines to be present.

■ Offer emotional support to both, acknowledging their different perspectives and enabling open and respectful discussion in a neutral space if possible.

■ Give detailed advice regarding the possible implications of the test results for Kay and offer a referral to a genetic counsellor for discussion about managing any potential results and coping with the potential impact on her daughter.

■ Give evidence-based information in a way that is accessible to Kay about the heritable nature of some types of breast cancer.

■ Look at the National Genomic Test Directory to determine what tests are available to Kay, how to access them and how long the results may take.

■ Construct a three or four generation family tree to inform cascade testing for other family members if this becomes appropriate following receipt of Kay's results.

■ Respect Orla's right to decline genetic testing and appreciate that she may not want to know if Kay tests positive for a BRCA gene variant.

■ Revise her own knowledge of privacy and confidentiality guidelines related to sharing genetic information within families.

■ Consider a balanced approach to privacy when offering cascade testing to Orla's extended family. If Kay's test is positive for a BRCA gene variant, breast cancer within the family can be classified as 'familial information' regarding risk; no disclosure regarding Orla's diagnosis or Kay's genetic profile needs to be made when planning predictive testing for other relatives.

Significant results

The practical aspects of the testing process, combined with long wait times and anxiety about potential outcomes can be trying. Patients attending for genomic tests can also feel 'swamped' by the amount of information they are given.(Kirk et al., 2011, p.36). Receiving results, even if they are long awaited, can be difficult and results may be accompanied by additional information related to treatment and to sharing genomic information with others. This can cause patients and families to be faced with challenging decisions.

A genetic diagnosis can be life changing. Some conditions are also life-limiting and patients or parents may find this news overwhelming. Patients often experience feelings of guilt if they have had children at a time when they were unaware that they could pass on a heritable condition. Some diagnoses may have financial implications in terms of attending care appointments and absence from work. If a person is no longer able to work owing to poor health, this can impact on their personal identity and feelings of worth. Nurses can feel a responsibility for the emotional and psychological impact of giving results which may affect a person's health, family relationships and shared future. Local genomic medicine service alliances (GMSAs) can be a source of support for nurses.

Rare and undiagnosed conditions

A major challenge in genomic medicine is the feeling of causing distress and anxiety for patients and parents (Kirk et al., 2011). These feelings can be amplified when patients wait a long time for diagnostic test results and receive no definitive answer. Nurses must manage patient or parent expectations and patients should be aware that genomic test results often take longer than other medical tests (Joint Committee on Genomics in Medicine, 2019). Expected waiting times are published by the genomic laboratory hubs and different test panels take different lengths of time.

The recent Deciphering Developmental Disorders study identified molecular diagnoses for thousands of infants and children across the UK and Ireland living with previously undiagnosed developmental disorders (Wright et al., 2023). It is, however, more often the case that for rare genetic diseases the cause of a patient's symptoms is not determined. When an unusual presentation has a suspected genetic cause there is a known 'diagnostic gap' owing to biomedical complexities and the stage of development of the technologies available for rare disease investigation and a diagnosis cannot always be made (Wang et al., 2023, p.1). It is more difficult to diagnose developmental disorders of Black Caribbean and Black African ancestry owing to a lack of representation in genetic databases and ancestry-matched controls (Wright et al., 2023; Kapadia et al., 2022). This means that the health care team cannot offer precision therapies.

It is possible for a negative result to be reported when a pathogenic variant has not been recognised. This does not mean that the cause of symptoms is not genetic but that a specific condition has not yet been discovered. This may be frustrating for patients or parents who are struggling to understand a range of symptoms and how to cope with them. Neurodevelopmental disorders, abnormal growth, dysmorphic features, unusual behaviours and speech delay are common features of undiagnosed genetic disorders in infants, which can cause communication problems, dependence and high clinical need (Wright et al., 2023). For patients and families this can mean multiple health appointments and tests, such as EEGs, lumbar puncture or sleep studies for seizures. Parents can experience barriers and long waits to access overburdened services and they may have to advocate for their child and negotiate for referrals.

Whole genome sequencing can be an option when there is difficulty diagnosing a condition but the term 'whole genome sequencing' can be misleading, even for health care practitioners. It is important to be aware that virtual panels of genes may be used in clinical applications of WGS. This means that although the whole genome is sequenced, only those genes known to be associated with the patient's features are usually analysed. When a health care practitioner requests a test that is described as a WGS panel test, this does not usually mean that their whole genome has been checked, only those genes included on the panel (Health Education England, 2022).

The American Society of Human Genetics (Botkin et al., 2015) recommends targeted tests in preference to whole genome sequencing in children and adolescents to avoid problems created by gathering more data than needed, including incidental findings and variants of uncertain significance. They also recommend that parents be given the opportunity to decline to receive data on either of these occurrences before tests are performed to avoid later ethical dilemmas.

A rare condition is one that affects fewer than 1 in 2000 people (Morris et al., 2022). Professionals must work collaboratively to keep pace with the changing health care environment when caring for those with rare conditions (Greco and Salveson, 2009). Kirk et al. (2011) identified that a multidisciplinary approach and well-co-ordinated care is necessary for the effective implementation of genomics into UK health services to avoid 'fragmentation' of care between settings (p.15). However, patients accessing services such as physiotherapy, audiology and speech therapy often experience a lack of co-ordination between these services. The lack of co-ordinated care for those with rare disease and their families can impact on their physical and mental health, often alongside the added strain of a financial impact (Morris et al., 2022).

The burden of worry about a child's future, their education and the support they will need if they have a rare or undiagnosed genetic condition can be tough and it is important that parents' voices are heard. The Genetic Alliance UK syndromes without a name (SWAN – https://geneticalliance.org.uk/support-and-information/swan-uk-syndromes-without-a-name/) project supports children with undiagnosed genetic conditions and their families (Genetic Alliance, 2025). Their work ensures that families are included in research to improve knowledge related to rare conditions and quality of life for those living with them. These families are likely to have many shared feelings and experiences, and research can help to understand these experiences and to improve care as genomics technologies develop (Weller et al., 2022).

 Knowledge focus

What does SWAN or being undiagnosed mean?

SWAN stands for Syndromes Without A Name. It is not a diagnosis, but a term used when a child or young adult is believed to have a genetic condition, and testing has failed to identify a genetic cause.

Syndromes without a name are also referred to as undiagnosed genetic conditions, unknown genetic conditions and undiagnosed genetic disorders.

Children affected by a syndrome without a name can have a range of different symptoms and each child is likely to be affected differently. However, many SWAN children are described as having global developmental delay, learning and/or physical disabilities or complex medical needs (Genetic Alliance, 2025).

Hamilton and Bowers (2007) define 'genetic vulnerability' as individual or family concerns related to genetic information. This term reflects how family value systems and joint experiences contribute to the impact of information about the genome. This includes how information about individual or family risk is understood and how difficult decision making may be for families and this vulnerability must be taken into account to provide effective nursing care and to meet patient and family needs.

Incidental findings

If an alternative or additional condition is identified by tests for a suspected condition and a patient has consented to receiving results about incidental findings, this can lead to difficult conversations. For example, when polycystic kidney disease is suspected, it is possible that another inherited pathogenic kidney condition may be identified from the renal panel of tests. Sources of support include the MDT for challenging cases, GMSAs and genetic counsellors who can support nurses to manage challenging cases.

Variants of uncertain significance

Test results can also show variants of uncertain significance. This could be the discovery of a pathogenic variant about which nothing is known. When there is no evidence base, it is difficult to make clinical decisions for variants of uncertain significance, which can cause frustration for patients or parents. Living with uncertainty about the present and the future can cause emotional distress for those who have invested hope in a diagnosis. Other challenges include the identification of genetic conditions for which there is little or no treatment available (Kirk et al., 2011). Again, nurses must manage expectations prior to tests and be clear that an answer may not be found and that the promise of personalised medicine does not deliver for all.

Misattributed paternity

Misattributed or 'false' paternity can also be flagged by genetic testing. This is when a man is believed by himself and others to be the biological father of a child, but it is discovered through genetic tests that he is not (Tozzo et al., 2014, p177). If a child is diagnosed with a genetic condition, confirmatory carrier testing may be offered to support their diagnosis. These tests identify carriers to address any implications for their own health and for the rest of the family. If a condition is identified in a child for which both parents must be carriers (for example an autosomal recessive condition), and the person who believes he is the father of the child is not a carrier for the condition, this will be revealed by confirmatory tests.

This information can cause upset and affect relationships. Deontological or moral debate has considered whether health care professionals have a duty to disclose misattributed paternity and if so, to whom they should disclose it. In the US, recommendations for pre-test counselling include information about the possibility of misattributed parentage through testing. It is recommended that health professionals do not disclose any misattributed parentage identified unless there is a clear clinical benefit that outweighs any potential psychological harm (ASHG, 2015).

It is helpful to have comprehensive and open discussions about both intended and incidental information which may be revealed by any test and to record preferences for each family member receiving information prior to testing (Tozzoet al., 2014).

Culturally competent care

It is essential that nurses have the skills to navigate cultural issues which arise in relation to genomics. Part of the nursing role is to meet community needs, and they should ask about and record a person's ethnicity and understand what this means in relation to the practices of local cultural and religious communities (Kirk et al., 2011). Some cultural practices mean that genetic risk is increased for some groups and the Health and Social Care Act (UK Government, 2012) affirms nurses' legal duty to help reduce health inequality.

Genomics incorporates risks to health from inherited genetic variations and from environmental factors and environmental risk can also be increased by cultural or lifestyle factors such as diet. Nurses are required to take accurate family histories and to discuss a person's lifestyle choices in order to recognise risks to health. They must build trusting relationships to facilitate obtaining relevant information and to support individuals and families to reduce risk.

Sometimes cultural practices can raise ethical questions which are difficult for nurses to navigate. Consanguineous (or close relative marriage) is practised in some communities in the UK and this practice greatly increases the risk of pathogenic congenital anomalies and genetic variants (for genetic conditions like cystic fibrosis) recurring within the same family. In order to support families, nurses must respect diverse cultural values and patient autonomy. Information can be provided relating to risk without judgement or blame. Members of many communities in the UK experience racism or Islamophobia. Some genetic conditions may also lead to stigmatisation. This can negatively impact those who need the most support, for example families and communities who practise consanguinity and have multiple experiences of baby loss.

These issues create an imperative for nurses to know their local communities and any inherent risks, and to understand the health beliefs of the patients they care for and the cultural implications of tests, diagnosis or treatment. Nurses can raise awareness of genetic and genomic risks to health using effective evidence-based approaches, for example acknowledging studies that highlight the less common use of technologies such as apps in ethnic minority groups (Kapadia et al., 2022). Accessibility of screening services can be improved by considering opening times and privacy or welcoming those who wish to be accompanied by friends or relatives. Skills for effective health promotion and education should be developed to meet the needs of those with all levels of health literacy. Medical terms can be difficult for most people to process but even more so in a different language and the use interpreters where necessary can make a positive difference (Kapadia et al., 2022).

Genomics and insurance

Genetic diagnoses can be a cause for financial anxiety, especially in the US where there is no national health system and people pay for health care and health insurance. Health care professionals practising genomic medicine have a duty to protect a person from discrimination based on their genetic information but insurance coverage for screening and treatment is unbalanced, creating a challenge for patients and for nurses in genetic services (Radford et al., 2014).

America has a Genetic Information Non-discrimination Act (GINA), which provides health insurance protections. Insurers cannot ask for genetic information about person or their family, including any genetic or genomic tests they have had, or use this information to determine coverage (United States Congress, 2008). GINA also prevents employers from using genetic information to make decisions about a person's employment, providing protection against discrimination, although it is often not appreciated that businesses with fewer than 15 employees are exempt from GINA regulations (Tluczek et al., 2019).

Alongside the provision of diagnostic data, the improved *predictive* capabilities of genetic testing pose challenges related to health and life insurance. Predicting future health through genetic testing has created some undesirable consequences, including the increased cost of insurance to cover all possible diseases linked with all identified variants despite the reality that some may never manifest. A predictive risk of Huntington's disease means that life insurance premiums will increase but that a person may not develop this condition. Health prediction is not always straightforward and context, often not included in insurance calculations, is important. Nurses can help people to reduce risk factors such as smoking but there remains inherent discrimination in using genetic data to increase cost because people cannot change their genes.

Insurance companies can use polygenic risk scoring to calculate actuarial risk and include this in the cost of insurance. They can also include pharmacogenomic data related to any likely reduced response to medication, for example owing to an identified liver enzyme deficiency. Increasing costs based on prediction and not reality is prejudicial (Dixon et al., 2023). The UK genetic testing code of practice, reviewed in 2018, includes the principle that insurers should not require diagnostic or predictive genetic tests to obtain insurance (UK Government, 2018A).

Health inequality

Differences in socioeconomic status, education and ethnic or cultural background create regions in every country where populations are underserved by health services (Tluczek et al., 2019). In addition to the many positive developments, for example in cancer care, provided by genomics, these disparities can be exacerbated. Some ethnic groups are at increased risk for inherited pathogenic variants and there may be a specific risk within a local community. Black women are more at risk from inherited TP53 mutations which affect DNA repair and can lead to aggressive endometrial cancers at a younger age, and those of Jewish descent are at increased risk from inheriting BRCA gene faults.

Equality, diversity and inclusion is a central facet of care, but it is widely acknowledged that for some, barriers to testing and treatment exacerbate ethnic health inequalities. Cultural, psychological and practical barriers mean that some ethnic groups access care less often than others. These barriers include a lack of knowledge about services, fear of discrimination, distrust of health care providers, a lack of access to interpreters, the inability to access digital services and a feeling that health services are detached from the communities they serve (Kapadia et al., 2022). Such factors can be addressed by working closely with local communities to meet their needs. Nursing efforts can contribute to ensuring equal access to specialists and resources by eliciting and addressing concerns, advocating for vulnerable groups and facilitating access to genomic tests (Kirk et al., 2011). Risk assessment and relevant preventive strategies linked with cultural norms and public education taking into account community values can improve local health (Allen, 2018).

Ethnicity is important in genomics, but individual ancestry can be complex. Two people who include themselves within one ethnic group may be genomically different and it is genomic heritage which can affect a person's level of risk for a heritable condition. Genetic polymorphisms or common gene variants affecting liver enzyme synthesis and activity also influence individual responses to medicines with increased prevalence of specific polymorphisms and reduced drug metabolism in some ethnic groups. For example, the BNF recommends pre-treatment screening prior to prescribing carbamazepine for individuals of Han Chinese or Thai origin. It is therefore necessary to ask and record ethnicity, but adding context can unintentionally influence how patients are cared for, for example unconscious bias can affect how health care practitioners give information.

Less is understood about genomics in some ethnicities than in others for example when calculating polygenic risk, which is explored in the previous chapter. Ethnic minority groups are also often reluctant to be involved in research to increase this understanding (Kapadia et al., 2022). Such projects include the Infant Mortality Task Force implemented to improve disparities in maternity care and wider societal issues impacting on maternal health to improve outcomes in Birmingham. This task force was formed following a report urging health care practitioners to identify opportunities to enhance genetic literacy and increase access to genetic services (Khan and Salway, 2020). Genomic data from the Born in Bradford study, started in 2007, also contributes to research on childhood disease the in UK. This study is multi-ethnic pregnancy and birth cohort study to establish determinants of health and development through life in a deprived population (Bird et al., 2019).

The ethical principle of justice (Beauchamp and Childress, 2001), which supports fair distribution and equitable use of resources, requires nurses to protect patients' universal rights for equal access to available care and technologies. Nurses are uniquely positioned to identify opportunities to address health disparities and should work to demonstrate inter-professional leadership and to integrate change into local policy (Tluczek et al., 2019).

📖 Learning activity – making balanced decisions

- Consider examples where each of the Beauchamp and Childress (2001) principles of biomedical ethics – beneficence, non-maleficence, justice and autonomy – might help nurses to make decisions related to genomic testing and ongoing patient care.

(This learning activity is linked to NHS England (2023) genomic nursing competency 5.)

Pre-natal genomic tests

Nursing skills include advocating for patients and supporting informed choices. If first trimester screening shows increased risk of a genetic disorder, nurses can request that a diagnostic test is prioritised. This might be obtaining genetic material from chorionic villus sampling or amniocentesis, looking for abnormalities via ultrasound scan or non-invasive pre-natal testing (explored in Chapter 4).

Consent for pre-natal genetic tests is usually given by the mother and requires careful consideration of the implications for the pregnancy if a genetic condition is found (Joint Committee on Genomics in Medicine, 2019). Parents may decide not to continue with a pregnancy following foetal diagnosis of disorders such as Down syndrome. If information from tests might affect the outcome of a pregnancy, nurses may face moral qualms regarding their actions. Pre-natal diagnosis raises some ethical concerns related to normalising screening and termination and lowering the incidence of certain conditions within a population. New treatments to increase bone growth for children born with achondroplasia, the most common form of dwarfism, have raised concerns from many people who believe that it should not be regarded as a condition that needs to be 'fixed' (Saner, 2020). It has also been posited that screening for some conditions attaches a value assumption to them regarding a reduced quality of life for those who are born with them (Newson, 2008).

There are important religious considerations for Muslims regarding the timing of a termination of pregnancy so tests must be performed as early as possible (Al-Matary and Ali, 2014). For personal or cultural reasons, some mothers may not wish to involve persons close to them in the decision to terminate a pregnancy and will require accurate information, time to make an informed choice and compassion. Women from ethnic groups may be concerned about staff imposing their own values upon them and nurses must be careful to provide culturally competent pre-natal care (Kapadia et al., 2022). Nurses can contact their local GMSA for support from genetic counsellors and reproductive advice.

Reproductive choices

Strategies to prevent a child from inheriting a genetic variant can be discussed when planning a pregnancy but there can be associated ethical issues. The 'designer babies' debate centres around the modification of the conception process to prevent a genetic condition and some groups view the management of human reproduction in this way as 'playing God' (Rossant, 2018). Nevertheless, IVF can be used to select healthy embryos if there is a heritable condition such as Lynch syndrome within a family. This method can also be used to determine the sex of an embryo, prior to implantation, to avoid conditions linked to variations in genes within the sex chromosomes, such as haemophilia.

Whole genome sequencing in newborns

Newborn genomic sequencing (nGS) can confer many benefits, including the early identification of actionable adult-onset diseases such as degenerative conditions and some cancers. Newborn screening programmes around the world include Baby Beyond in Australia and BabySeq, based in Boston, USA. The Genomics England 'Generation Study' is focused on conditions meeting specific criteria including a range of metabolic, immune system or thyroid conditions which appear before age 5 that can be treated with medication, dietary changes or bone marrow transplant. Detection of a condition before it manifests can greatly improve outcomes (Wilkinson, 2023). This type of testing can also have benefits for families; if a heritable BRCA gene mutation is identified, the child will not be at immediate risk but both parents can seek individual risk assessments (Botkin and Rothwell, 2016).

The UK media reports on the significant benefits of newborn genomic screening for improving future national health and care. However, concerns that parents joining the programme may not understand all possible consequences of the tests have led to challenges about whether 'robust' consent is consistently obtained (Horton et al., 2015, p.1). This could be a result of ineffective education or a lack of information being given to the parents of newborns participating in this research (Botkin and Rothwell, 2016). Parents may be keen to sign up and realise potential benefits while not appreciating the significance of all possible outcomes and the potential for associated distress and feelings of guilt or blame if a genetic risk to their child's health is identified (Pereira et al., 2021).

Additional ethical concerns surround the psychosocial impact of receiving results when for some, trauma may be caused unnecessarily. Newborn genomic screening includes multiple assays to test for rare genetic conditions, but variants identified by these tests which initially cause concern can prove to be insignificant. Competing challenges include cost but the biggest ethical opposition to newborn screening stems from the potential for harm caused by false positive results (Botkin and Rothwell, 2016). Variants associated with some diseases, for example the TMYBPC3 gene variant associated with hypertrophic cardiomyopathy, can appear in healthy adults. Not all carriers of the implicated variant go on to develop a cardiomyopathy and some individuals will carry such variants throughout their lives and never develop a condition. Their quality of life however, may be negatively affected by the knowledge that they could begin to experience symptoms at any time (Dixon et al., 2023).

Tests may also identify heritable variants for a condition which the child will go on to develop but for which there is no benefit to early intervention. Existing treatments may be prohibitively expensive or not proven to be effective, causing parental distress. On occasion, genomic tests can raise questions about the future management of any conditions identified. Issues raised and the resulting psychological harm may outweigh the intended benefits (Horton et al., 2024). Broader ethical concerns include performing tests, the results of which may significantly affect their future choices, on babies who cannot consent for themselves (Wilkinson, 2023).

Significantly, however, a US clinical trial measuring psychosocial impact when an increased health risk is identified via nGS found no lasting impact on parent–child relationships, strain on the parents' relationship or on parental distress, including postpartum depression (Pereira et al., 2021). These findings provide reassurance as whole genome screening in newborns contributes to research that enables scientists to map sequence variations affecting disease severity and response to treatment. This assists with better understanding and characterisation of conditions and supports the continued development of personalised medicine (Botkin and Rothwell, 2016). Such research can also lead to the identification of new conditions and determine how information from the genome might be used across a person's lifespan (Wilkinson, 2023).

Many parents decline to participate in nGS, giving reasons such as a lack of interest in research and discomfort with genetic testing. Also reported is anxiety concerning privacy and confidentiality and regarding future health insurance if a condition or uncertain results were to be identified and included in their family medical records. Understanding parental perceptions of testing and addressing and validating concerns may help to facilitate discussion when approaching parents for consent (Genetti et al., 2019).

Responsible and ethical research

The Ethical, Legal and Social Implications research programme, formed as part of the Human Genome Project (1990–2003), recognised that WGS would raise ethical concerns, for example those related to consent and privacy. Those participating in research and giving access to their genetic data must be able to provide informed consent and a separate part of the NHS (2021) consent form for patients consenting to a genomic test records their additional consent to contribute to the National Genomic Research Library. Those consenting must receive information about how their information will be used, stored and protected and there is a webpage about this for them (Genomics England, 2024).

Research institutions, universities and pharmaceutical companies can access the genetic and health information in the national genetic database (Wilkinson, 2023). Patients must be informed about any potential risks and should understand that participation is voluntary. They should know that they can withdraw from the study at any time and what will happen to their data or samples in this instance. Protection of participant data is carefully regulated, and nurses involved in conducting research must demonstrate understanding of guidelines.

Researchers will plan for incidental findings as part of studies. This can be challenging because such findings are not always possible to predict. Researchers collecting genomic data related to a single phenomenon, such as heredity patterns in twin studies or family studies, may identify unexpected mutations known to cause adult-onset degenerative conditions like Huntington's disease. All participants should be given the opportunity to discuss what they would want to be disclosed to them in this instance and these preferences should be recorded. Importantly, patients should know that they can change their minds about receiving information related to incidental findings and opt out at a later stage (Sanderson et al., 2019). When considering the disclosure of findings, researchers should consider each situation as unique. The National Human Genome Research Institute specifies that researchers have a responsibility to report incidental findings if they can be validated, have health implications and will enable actions to be taken which may improve the person's health.

People managing genetic conditions, sometimes without a diagnosis, often have challenging lives. What is most important to them should be important to health care practitioners, but a clinical focus can lead to patients feeling overlooked as individuals. When conducting genomics research, researchers must take care to maintain a sense of identity by listening to and validating concerns. It is important to appreciate that individuals have different levels of understanding, and that people sometimes misunderstand or forget what they have given consent for. 'Risk' also means different things to different people, levels of risk are perceived differently and the feeling of being at risk impacts people in different ways (Nolan et al., 2024). Genetic Alliance UK is a group that advocates for those with rare diseases and carers to ensure their views are counted in the development of UK strategy. Some of their work involves supporting research in the NHS, including the Generation Study (Genetic Alliance UK, 2024).

Gene therapy

Gene therapy can improve the lives of some people with genetic conditions. The insertion of a functioning gene where there is a non-functioning variant can restore function and reduce the effects of a condition. Recent examples in the national media include successful treatment for angioedema, a painful genetic swelling disorder, with a single dose of Crispr-Cas9 (Richard Warry, BBC News, 2024). A permanent cure can be life-changing for many eligible patients. CRISPR genome editing technology has also been developed to treat bone cancer and graft treatments are being tested for future use (Your Genome, 2024). In 2023, the UK medicines and health care products regulatory agency (MHRA) approved Casgevy, the first gene editing treatment for transfusion-dependent beta-thalassaemia and sickle cell disease in patients over 12 years old (Parums, 2024).

Spinal muscular atrophy is an inherited, life-limiting neuromuscular disorder that affects motor neurons and causes progressive muscle wasting. It can develop in adults, and some babies are born with this condition. These babies can have difficulty feeding and swallowing, respiratory issues and developmental delay. Eligible infants under the age of 2 years may be treated effectively with gene therapy to restore nerve function with the provision of an unaffected gene (Euro GCT, 2024).

Gene therapy has many benefits but also carries a risk of harm as treatments are developed and trialled. Development is regulated, and a gene therapy advisory committee employs strict governance. Gene therapy medicinal products must be licensed as safe and effective prior to use (Specialist Pharmacy Service, 2024). The development of CRISPR technologies has sparked ethical concerns regarding the ability to generate heritable changes in the genome (Rossant, 2018).

There are also ethical concerns related to the potential for inequitable access to this technology. Some disquiet surrounds the excessive cost of genomic advances at a time when the National Health Service is struggling with recruitment and retention of staff (Wilkinson, 2023). However, the more genomic technologies evolve, the more useful they become with new discoveries consistently improving standards of care to reduce cost (Botkin and Rothwell, 2016).

Stem cell research

Human stem cells can help scientists to understand and to prevent genetic conditions. These cells can be grown from adult or embryo tissue samples and used to develop cells and tissues for transplant, for example, haematopoietic blood cells and bone marrow cells in the treatment of leukaemia. Stem cells can also be used to test the effects and possible toxicity of chemotherapy.

There are however ethical concerns related to obtaining cells from embryos and there are strict bioethics regulations for growing new tissues in laboratories. The Human Fertilisation and Embryology Authority (https://www.hfea.gov.uk/) is responsible for approving all UK stem cell research. Licensing conditions stipulate that this research is necessary:

- to increase knowledge about the causes of congenital disease;
- to develop methods for detecting the presence of gene or chromosome abnormalities;
- to increase knowledge about serious disease;
- to enable such knowledge to be applied in developing treatments for serious disease (University of Leicester, 2024).

Private or direct to consumer tests

Direct to consumer genomic tests can be accessed via the internet without consultation with a health professional. People can also buy direct to consumer pharmacogenomic tests. This has raised concerns about the 'unproven clinical validity or clinical utility' of the tests (Lea et al., 2011, p.7). Direct to consumer testing also raises questions about the ownership of cells and tissues once they have been submitted to the testing company.

There are concerns that patients buying tests online are not given adequate information or effective counselling prior to testing. Counselling from a health care practitioner is important to support people to receive any potential results and sometimes, after receiving their results, to make choices that are right for them (ASHG, 2015). Those accessing private genetic or genomic tests may need somebody to interpret the results and to explain their significance for them and their families, but health professionals should be cautious if they are asked to do this because there are high chances of inaccurate results (Royal College General Practitioners, 2019).

Summary
The genetic testing process can raise many ethical issues. The implications of testing for patients and their families and any ethical questions should be carefully considered prior to testing to achieve adequately informed consent. Ethical questions create challenges for nurses and advanced skills and knowledge are required to navigate these. There are guidelines, resources and sources of support for nurses including local GMSAs.

Nursing resources
- NHS England offers a free e-learning programme for health care practitioners which helps them to understand some of the issues associated with close relative or consanguineous marriage and to inform and improve care: https://www.e-lfh.org.uk/programmes/close-relative-marriage/
- Detailed case examples followed by guidance on how to manage them ethically are included in the Royal College of Physicians guidance (Joint committee on genomics in medicine, 2019): www.rcplondon.ac.uk/projects/outputs/consent-and-confidentiality-genomic-medicine
- Helix of Love is a collection of poems produced as part of the 'Ethical Preparedness in Genomic Medicine' project, funded by the Wellcome trust. The poems offer insight to those caring for people and families affected by rare genetic conditions: https://www.bsms.ac.uk/research/clinical-and-experimental-medicine/theoretical-and-empirical-bioethics/helix-of-love.aspx

Resources for patients
- The Health Centre for Genomics Education in NSW Australia has a video to support discussion about genomic tests and a downloadable factsheet for patients to read prior to testing: https://www.health.nsw.gov.au/services/Factsheets/genomic-testing-patient-factsheet.pdf
- EuroStemCell is a network of scientists and academics who provide educational resources for the public and for educational settings related to the use of stem cells in health care in a number of languages: https://www.eurostemcell.org/

References
ABC v. St George's Healthcare NHS Trust [2015] EWHC 1394 (QB); [2017] EWCA Civ 336 (CA).
Allen, D., 2018. Genetic Testing: how genetics and genomics can affect healthcare disparities. *Clinical Journal of Oncology Nursing*, 22(1), 116–118.

Al-Matary, A. and Ali, J., 2014. Controversies and considerations regarding the termination of pregnancy for foetal anomalies in Islam. *BMC Medical Ethics*, *15*, pp.1–10.

Beauchamp, T.L. and Childress, J.F., 2001. *Principles of Biomedical Ethics*. Oxford University Press, New York.

Bird, P.K., McEachan, R.R., Mon-Williams, M., Small, N., West, J., Whincup, P., Wright, J., Andrews, E., Barber, S.E., Hill, L.J. and Lennon, L., 2019. Growing up in Bradford: protocol for the age 7–11 follow up of the Born in Bradford birth cohort. *BMC Public Health*, *19*, pp.1–12.

Botkin, J.R. and Rothwell, E., 2016. Whole genome sequencing and newborn screening. *Current Genetic Medicine Reports*, *4*, pp.1–6.

Botkin, J.R., Belmont, J.W., Berg, J.S., Berkman, B.E., Bombard, Y., Holm, I.A., Levy, H.P., Ormond, K.E., Saal, H.M., Spinner, N.B. and Wilfond, B.S., 2015. Points to consider: ethical, legal, and psychosocial implications of genetic testing in children and adolescents. *The American Journal of Human Genetics*, *97*(1), pp.6–21.

Dixon, P., Horton, R., Newman, W.G., McDermott, J.H. and Lucassen, A., 2023. *Genomics and Insurance in the United Kingdom: Increasing Complexity and Emerging Challenges* (No. p3hsy). Center for Open Science.

Dove, E.S., Chico, V., Fay, M., Laurie, G., Lucassen, A.M. and Postan, E., 2019. Familial genetic risks: how can we better navigate patient confidentiality and appropriate risk disclosure to relatives? *Journal of Medical Ethics*, *45*(8), pp.504–507.

Euro GCT, 2024. What conditions can currently be treated using gene and stem cell therapy? https://www.eurogct.org/what-conditions-can-currently-be-treated-using-gene-and-cell-therapy (accessed 2 April 2024).

Genetic Alliance UK, 2024. Improving research and services. https://geneticalliance.org.uk/campaigns-and-research/improving-genomic-research-and-services/ (accessed 17 April 2024).

Genetic Alliance UK, 2025. SWAN UK. https://geneticalliance.org.uk/support-and-information/swan-uk-syndromes-without-a-name/ (accessed 11 March 2025).

Genetti, C.A., Schwartz, T.S., Robinson, J.O., VanNoy, G.E., Petersen, D., Pereira, S., Fayer, S., Peoples, H.A., Agrawal, P.B., Betting, W.N. and Holm, I.A., 2019. Parental interest in genomic sequencing of newborns: enrollment experience from the BabySeq Project. *Genetics in Medicine*, *21*(3), pp.622–630.

Genomics England, 2024. How your data is used. https://www.genomicsengland.co.uk/patients-participants/data/ (accessed 23 April 2024).

Greco, K.E. and Salveson, C., 2009. Identifying genetics and genomics nursing competencies common among published recommendations. *Journal of Nursing Education*, *48*(10), pp.557–565.

Hamilton, R. J. and Bowers, B.J., 2007. The theory of genetic vulnerability: a Roy model exemplar. *Nursing Science Quarterly*, *20*(3), 254–264.

Health Education, England 2021. Facilitating genomic testing: a competency framework. https://www.genomicseducation.hee.nhs.uk/wp-content/uploads/2021/06/Facilitiating-genomic-testing-competencies-final.pdf

Health Education England, 2022. Whole genome sequencing. https://www.genomicseducation.hee.nhs.uk/genotes/knowledge-hub/whole-genome-sequencing/ (accessed 22 April 2024).

Horton, R., Wright, C.F., Firth, H.V., Turnbull, C., Lachmann, R., Houlston, R.S. and Lucassen, A., 2024. Challenges of using whole genome sequencing in population newborn screening. *bmj*, *384*. https://doi.org/10.1136/bmj-2023-077060

Joint Committee on Genomics in Medicine, 2019. Consent and confidentiality on genomic medicine. Royal College of physicians: London. www.rcplondon.ac.uk/projects/outputs/consent-and-confidentiality-genomic-medicine (accessed 11 March 2024).

Kapadia, D., Zhang, J., Salway, S., Nazroo, J., Booth, A., Villarroel-Williams, N., Becares, L. and Esmail, A., 2022. Ethnic inequalities in healthcare: a rapid evidence review. https://www.nhsrho.org/wp-content/uploads/2023/05/RHO-Rapid-Review-Final-Report_.pdf

Khan, N. and Salway, S., 2022. Communities that prefer close blood marriages need more help to access genetic services. https://blogs.bmj.com/bmj/2020/02/12/communities-that-prefer-close-blood-marriages-need-more-help-to-access-genetic-services/ (accessed 3 April 2024).

Kirk, M., Campalani, S., Doris, F., Heron, J., Mannion, G., Metcalfe, A., Patch, C., Permalloo, N., Shepherd, M. and Calzone, K., 2011. Genetics/genomics in nursing and midwifery: Task and Finish Group report to the Nursing and Midwifery Professional Advisory Board. https://assets.publishing.service.gov.uk/media/5a7cb326ed915d63cc65c50d/dh_131947.pdf

Lea, D.H., Skirton, H., Read, C.Y. and Williams, J.K., 2011. Implications for educating the next generation of nurses on genetics and genomics in the 21st century. *Journal of Nursing Scholarship*, 43(1), pp.3–12

Morris, S., Hudson, E., Bloom, L., Chitty, L.S., Fulop, N.J., Hunter, A., Jones, J., Kai, J., Kerecuk, L., Kokocinska, M. and Leeson-Beevers, K., 2022. Co-ordinated care for people affected by rare diseases: the CONCORD mixed-methods study. *Health and Social Care Delivery Research*, 10(5), pp.1–220.

National Data Guardian, 2020. The eight Caldicott principles. https://assets.publishing.service.gov.uk/media/5fcf9b92d3bf7f5d0bb8bb13/Eight_Caldicott_Principles_08.12.20.pdf

Newson, A.J., 2008, April. Ethical aspects arising from non-invasive foetal diagnosis. *Seminars in Fetal and Neonatal Medicine*, 13(2), pp.103–108.

NHS (2021) NHS Genomics Medicine Service record of discussion form. https://www.england.nhs.uk/wp-content/uploads/2021/09/nhs-genomic-medicine-service-record-of-discussion-form.pdf (accessed 29 May 2025).

NHS England, 2021. Record of discussion form. https://www.england.nhs.uk/publication/nhs-genomic-medicine-service-record-of-discussion-form/

NHS England, 2023. The 2023 genomic competency framework for UK nurses. https://www.genomicseducation.hee.nhs.uk/wp-content/uploads/2023/12/2023-Genomic-Competency-Framework-for-UK-Nurses.pdf

Nicol, M.J., 2002. The teaching of genetics in New Zealand undergraduate nursing programmes. *Nurse Education Today*, 22(5), pp.401–408.

Nolan, J.J., Forrest, J. and Ormondroyd, E., 2024. Additional findings from the 100,000 Genomes Project: a qualitative study of recipient perspectives. *Genetics in Medicine*, 26(6), p.101103.

Parums, D.V., 2024. First regulatory approvals for CRISPR-Cas9 therapeutic gene editing for sickle cell disease and transfusion-dependent β-thalassemia. *Medical Science Monitor: International Medical Journal of Experimental and Clinical Research*, 30, pp.e944204-1.

Pereira, S., Smith, H.S., Frankel, L.A., Christensen, K.D., Islam, R., Robinson, J.O., Genetti, C.A., Zawatsky, C.L.B., Zettler, B., Parad, R.B. and Waisbren, S.E., 2021. Psychosocial effect of newborn genomic sequencing on families in the BabySeq Project: a randomized clinical trial. *JAMA Pediatrics*, 175(11), pp.1132–1141.

Radford, C., Prince, A., Lewis, K. and Pal, T., 2014. Factors which impact the delivery of genetic risk assessment services focused on inherited cancer genomics: expanding the role and reach of certified genetics professionals. *Journal of Genetic Counseling*, 23, pp.522–530.

Rossant, J., 2018. Gene editing in human development: ethical concerns and practical applications. *Development*, 145(16), p.dev150888.

Royal College General Practitioners, 2019. Genomic position statement. https://www.rcgp.org.uk/representing-you/policy-areas/genomic-position-statement (accessed 25 October 2024).

Sanderson, S.C., Lewis, C., Patch, C., Hill, M., Bitner-Glindzicz, M. and Chitty, L.S., 2019. Opening the 'black box' of informed consent appointments for genome sequencing: a multisite observational study. *Genetics in Medicine*, 21(5), pp.1083–1091.

Saner, 2020. 'There is a fear that this will eradicate dwarfism': the controversy over a new growth drug. https://www.theguardian.com/science/2020/sep/28/there-is-a-fear-that-this-will-eradicate-dwarfism-the-controversy-over-a-new-growth-drug

Specialist Pharmacy Service, 2024. Pan UK Pharmacy Working Group for ATMPs Gene Therapy Medicinal Products Governance and Preparation Requirements version 3. https://www.sps.nhs.uk/wp-content/uploads/2024/02/PAN-UK-PWG-for-ATMPs-Gene-Therapy-Guidance-V3.pdf (accessed 14 April 2024).

Strategic Reform and Planning, 2021. Guidance for health professionals obtaining consent for clinical genomic testing genomic-testing-consent-guidance.pdf (nsw.gov.au) (accessed 26 April 2024).

Tluczek, A., Twal, M.E., Beamer, L.C., Burton, C.W., Darmofal, L., Kracun, M., Zanni, K.L. and Turner, M., 2019. How American Nurses Association Code of Ethics informs genetic/genomic nursing. *Nursing Ethics*, 26(5), pp.1505–1517.

Tozzo, P., Caenazzo, L. and Parker, M.J., 2014. Discovering misattributed paternity in genetic counselling: different ethical perspectives in two countries. *Journal of Medical Ethics*, 40(3), pp.177–181.

UK Government, 2004. Human Tissue Act. https://www.legislation.gov.uk/ukpga/2004/30/contents (accessed April 2024).

UK Government, 2005. Mental Capacity Act 2005. https://www.legislation.gov.uk/ukpga/2005/9/contents/enacted (accessed April 2024)

UK Government, 2012. Health and Social Care Act. https://www.legislation.gov.uk/ukpga/2012/7/contents (accessed April 2024).

UK Government, 2018A. Code on genetic testing and insurance. https://assets.publishing.service.gov.uk/media/5bd08dd1ed915d78af510220/code-on-genetic-testing-and-insurance.pdf (accessed 19 April 2024).

UK Government, 2018B. Data protection Act. Data Protection Act 2018. https://www.gov.uk/government/collections/data-protection-act-2018 (accessed 10 April 2024).

United States Congress, 2008. Genetic Information non-discrimination Act. https://www.congress.gov/110/plaws/publ233/PLAW-110publ233.pdf (accessed 10 April 2024).

University of Leicester, 2024. Genetics and law for higher education. https://le.ac.uk/vgec/topics/genetics-and-ethics-and-law/higher-education/law (accessed 7 March 2024).

Wang, R., Helbig, I., Edmondson, A.C., Lin, L. and Xing, Y., 2023. Splicing defects in rare diseases: transcriptomics and machine learning strategies towards genetic diagnosis. *Briefings in Bioinformatics*, 24(5), p.bbad284.

Warry, R., BBC News 2024 Angiodema: gene therapy blocks painful hereditary disorder. https://www.bbc.com/news/health-68164372 (accessed 23 March 2024).

Weller, S., Lyle, K. and Lucassen, A., 2022. Re-imagining 'the patient': linked lives and lessons from genomic medicine. *Social Science & Medicine*, 297, p.114806.

Wilkinson, E., 2023. Newborn genome screening: a step too far. *The Pharmaceutical Journal*. https://pharmaceutical-journal.com/article/feature/newborn-genome-screening-a-step-too-far (accessed 23 March 2024).

Wright, C.F., Campbell, P., Eberhardt, R.Y., Aitken, S., Perrett, D., Brent, S., Danecek, P., Gardner, E.J., Chundru, V.K., Lindsay, S.J. and Andrews, K., 2023. Genomic diagnosis of rare pediatric disease in the United Kingdom and Ireland. *New England Journal of Medicine*, 388(17), pp.1559–1571.

Your Genome, 2024. Applications of Gene therapy. https://www.yourgenome.org/theme/applications-of-gene-therapy/ (accessed 4 April 2024).

Pharmacogenomics

Chapter outline

Pharmacogenomics is concerned with how an individual's genes can determine their response to medicines. Individuals may have common genetic variants or polymorphisms which can affect either their response to a specific drug or how their body processes certain groups of drugs, increasing the risk of medicines related harm. Nurses have a professional responsibility for protecting patients from avoidable harm and personalised care must incorporate medicines safety. Pre-treatment pharmacogenetic and pharmacogenomic testing is becoming more widely available and this can help those who prescribe, administer and monitor responses to medications to predict and minimise risks to achieve safer care and better outcomes.

Introduction

The safe administration of medication including monitoring medication effects to prevent harm where possible and to optimise treatment benefits is an integral part of the nursing role (Hetland et al., 2024). The role of the nurse in avoiding medicines related harms is expanding as many nurses are becoming independent and supplementary prescribers. These nurses must understand how drugs work, how the body processes drugs and both drug-specific and patient factors which have the potential to affect pharmacological action (Lea et al., 2011). Pharmacogenomics is a domain of pharmacology that focuses on individual genetic and genomic factors and the associated effects on patient responses to a wide range of medicines.

Different people can take the same drug with very different outcomes. Variability in the effectiveness of many commonly prescribed medicines has previously been attributed to prescribing factors such as dose, in combination with individual factors such

DOI: 10.4324/9781003453048-7

as patient age, adherence, comorbidities or interactions with the other medicines they take. It is now recognised that genetic makeup can also affect individual responses to many drugs (McDermott and Newman, 2023). This understanding means that it is sometimes possible to predict and prevent harmful responses to medicines in some individuals, reducing negative outcomes and the huge cost to the NHS of preventable adverse drug reactions (ADRs) (Royal College of Physicians and British Pharmacological Society, 2022).

It is estimated that up to 95% of the UK population carry at least one common gene variant or single nucleotide polymorphism (SNP) which can alter their response to a drug by affecting pharmacokinetic processes or how the body handles the drug (van der Wouden et al., 2020). Polymorphisms can also increase risks related to a drug's pharmacodynamic action or the effects the drug has on the body. These risks can be avoided by identifying any polymorphisms which have the potential to cause harmful reactions such as drug action at unintended sites (side effects) owing to ineffective metabolism or breakdown leading to an accumulation of the drug in the blood plasma. The terms pharmacogenetics and pharmacogenomics are often used interchangeably but pharmacogenomics has more emphasis on the influence of the whole genome on drug response (Rahma et al., 2020; Hetland et al., 2024).

Adverse responses to medicines can be multifactorial, involving variations in one or more genes plus patient factors such as age and environmental or lifestyle influences that can affect how the body processes them (Yousseff et al., 2020). Pharmacogenetic information can help prescribers to identify risk and prioritise safety, for example by avoiding particular drugs or adjusting the dose, or through effective monitoring for specific individuals (Taylor et al., 2020). In addition to safety benefits, tailoring both drug and dose to a patient's genotype can improve therapeutic outcomes and reduce costs from prescribing ineffective drugs. Pharmacogenomic tests currently contribute to safer care for many patients who have been prescribed a range of medicines and all members of the interprofessional health care team are now required to develop an understanding of how genomic technology can support effective care (Cheek, 2017).

⚑ Professional guidance: safe medicines administration

In order to administer medicines safely, all health care professionals, including nurses must:

- assess suitability and inherent risk for patient self-administration of medication;
- if medication is to be administered, administer medications in accordance with a valid prescription or other legal mechanism of supply for which they are deemed competent;
- be appropriately trained, assessed as competent and meet professional and regulatory standards;
- be accountable for actions and omissions, exercising professionalism and professional judgement at all times;
- follow agreed local processes and make necessary checks to avoid the risk of harm;
- have knowledge about each medicine to be administered including clinical indication, side effects and other relevant safety information;
- calculate drug doses accurately and in accordance with product guidance;

- give information regarding risk and obtain informed consent, performing an assessment of capacity to give consent when necessary;
- keep accurate and timely records of administration and omission;
- monitor the effects of medication and report and manage adverse drug reactions appropriately and in accordance with local policy (Royal Pharmaceutical Society, 2019).

Pharmacodynamics

Whether prescribing, administering, or monitoring the effects of a medication nurses have a responsibility to understand the causes of potential harms. Drugs act at intended and at unintended targets within the body to create both therapeutic and adverse effects. It is important for nurses to ascertain whether a medicine is working to manage the condition or symptoms it was prescribed for and to ask patients about any other effects they are experiencing following medication administration (Nursing and Midwifery Council, 2018). Nurses can help to ensure a patient knows when they should start to feel that their medicine is working, what to do if they feel it is not working and who to tell if they are experiencing any unexpected symptoms since starting a new medication. The most common types of medication side effects are Type A drug reactions, which are predictable from a drug's pharmacology, and Type B allergic or sensitivity type reactions (Coulson, 2021). The likelihood of experiencing both of these types of adverse response to a drug can be affected by a person's genetic makeup.

Medicines optimisation is a common goal for health care practitioners and four key principles can help them to maximise benefits and to minimise the risks associated with medicines (Royal Pharmaceutical Society, 2013). Understanding patient experiences related to their medicines regimes, making evidence-based treatment choices, prioritising medicines safety and following these principles routinely can help nurses to identify (and discuss the discontinuation of) medications not creating the desired effects or medicines creating harmful effects. It is estimated that for many drugs used to treat a range of conditions only 50–75% of patients experience a beneficial response (Taylor et al., 2020). Routine medicines review should include a structured examination of a person's medicines regime to try to optimise impact and minimise problems for individuals (NICE, 2015). Consideration of pharmacogenomic factors which can help optimise medicines use for individuals can contribute to the overall medicines' safety agenda within UK health care. Pharmacogenomics and Medicines optimisation comprise one of the NHS Genomics Networks of Excellence, to support progress in these areas within the NHS (NHS England, 2024). All nurses working with medicinal products and devices are responsible for medicines safety and should be aware of current progress towards the implementation of pharmacogenomic testing and developments which support routine access to and the use of test results within patient care pathways.

Pharmacokinetics

Genetically influenced variations in the way the body handles drugs can cause the plasma concentration of a drug to be too low or too high. Drug absorption, distribution, metabolism and excretion comprise processes that determine whether adequate amounts of drug reach the blood plasma, are carried to the target site and remain in the plasma for long enough to exert the required therapeutic effect. Changes to these processes can also decrease drug biotransformation or breakdown and elimination, creating the potential for an accumulation of drug in the body and potentially harmful effects within body systems (McGavock, 2017).

Pharmacogenomic variation most commonly affects the metabolic phase of drug elimination. Some drugs are subject to Phase 1 metabolism, which prepares them for elimination or permanent removal from the body. This is a destructive process where the cytochrome P450 or CYP450 enzyme family biotransforms a drug into its metabolites or chemically simpler substances which the body can excrete, usually in the urine (McGavock, 2017). Disease, other drugs and genetic SNPs can all affect the production and function of liver enzymes responsible for metabolising particular drugs for clearance. Variations to the genes involved in processing medicines, or pharmacogenes, can produce variations in enzyme activity and how individuals metabolise medicines. Single nucleotide polymorphisms most commonly affect the action of the CYP450 (cytochrome P450) enzymes in the liver, which break down most commonly prescribed drugs (Youssef et al., 2020). Reduced metabolism often results in larger quantities of drug than are required (a supratherapeutic plasma concentration), which increases the risk of adverse effects.

It is important to ask patients about any previous drug reactions or known polymorphisms when taking a medication history. Nurses are also instrumental in maintaining patient safety by letting patients know about any new symptoms or adverse effects they should report. When discussing treatment options, nurses should be equipped with adequate knowledge to ensure that patients are fully informed about any inherent risks. For example, some liver enzymes are responsible for transforming drugs into their active forms and if a person has a CYP2C19 enzyme deficiency, they may be unable to achieve therapeutic levels of drugs such as clopidogrel. Clopidogrel is prescribed to prevent platelet aggregation following a thrombotic event. This drug is an inactive precursor or pro-drug which must be bio-transformed into the substance which can exert a pharmacodynamic action. Low or subtherapeutic plasma levels of the clinically active metabolites of clopidogrel could lead to a thrombus and increase the patient's risk of experiencing a stroke (Lea et al., 2011).

Metaboliser status is determined by pharmacogenetic variations within the CYP450 enzyme family. Individuals can be categorised in relation to the level of function of specific CYP enzymes:

- poor metabolisers – little to no enzyme activity;
- intermediate metabolisers – decreased enzyme activity (activity between normal and poor metabolisers);
- normal metabolisers – fully functional enzyme activity;
- rapid metabolisers – increased enzyme activity compared with normal metabolisers but less than ultrarapid metabolisers;
- ultra-rapid metabolisers – increased enzyme activity compared with rapid metabolisers.

These terms describe relative levels of enzyme activity and are definitions that have been reached by expert consensus to provide clarity for prescribers (Caudle et al., 2017). The term 'phenotype' is used to denote the specific type of polymorphism a person has.

For example, a person with a lower than normal but still active level of CYP2C19 enzyme activity may be described as having an intermediate CYP2C19 metaboliser phenotype. Individuals with the more extreme phenotypes (poor or ultra-rapid) are most at risk of drug toxicities (Clark, 2020).

Awareness of phenotype and pharmacogenomic considerations enables prescribers to adjust doses appropriately or to avoid specific drugs that may not reach effective plasma levels. For poor metabolisers of CYP2C19 with little or no enzyme activity, ticagrelor can be used as an unlicensed alternative to clopidogrel (Royal College of Physicians and British Pharmacological Society, 2022). A DNA sample, provided by a simple buccal swab prior to the prescription of clopidogrel, can be used to identify CYP2C19 poor metaboliser phenotypes who have CYP2C19*2 variants leading to a loss of function of this enzyme (Cheek, 2017). NICE (2024B) has recently produced guidance to guide antiplatelet therapy following ischaemic stroke, although CYP2C19 testing is not currently widely available in the UK (NICE, 2024A).

Codeine

Understanding the effects of polymorphisms can help to determine appropriate dose, for example for fast or slow metabolisers of codeine (Lea et al., 2011). Codeine, commonly prescribed for pain relief, is another example of a pro-drug that must be metabolised by liver enzymes into an active form. This biotransformation is mediated by the CYP2D6 enzyme which belongs to the CYP450 enzyme superfamily. One of the active metabolites of codeine is morphine (M6G or morphine-6-glucuronide) and it is this metabolite that creates an analgesic effect.

Skills focus – standards for the assessment and management of pain

In order to provide effective care when working with those experiencing acute and chronic pain, nurses must have the skills to know when switching drugs or adjusting dose is necessary. Nurses must:

- be able to assess pain and deliver evidence-based pain management;
- be familiar with comprehensive and consistent pain assessment using valid and reliable tools;
- work collaboratively within the multi-disciplinary team; and
- recognise the boundaries of their clinical competence and seek advice as required (Cox et al., 2015).

Nurses must communicate well with patients to determine the clinical efficacy of any medications administered and then liaise with prescribers if necessary. Patients with fast or slow metaboliser phenotypes might not be aware of this trait at the time of medication administration. An indicator of a potential problem is a lack of therapeutic response even at the maximum recommended dose of drug. This could mean that little or no enzyme activity is producing little or no active drug metabolite, leading to insufficient analgesia. Lack of drug efficacy and the desired outcome can lead to a poor patient experience (Caudle et al., 2017).

Patients who are ultra-rapid CYP2D6 metabolisers transform codeine into morphine at an increased rate and to a larger extent. If these individuals are prescribed the recommended dose of codeine, they may be at risk of a supratherapeutic plasma concentration of morphine. Nurses should monitor the effects of codeine as routine to ensure that patients are receiving effective pain relief but also to identify morphine-related side effects and symptoms associated with morphine toxicity, such as drowsiness, confusion and breathing difficulties (Youssef et al., 2020).

❗ MHRA (2014) Safety alert: codeine and breastfeeding

Breastfed babies can rarely develop symptoms of toxicity owing to the presence of morphine in breast milk. This risk is associated with maternal codeine use for pain relief in ultra-rapid codeine metabolisers (resulting from CYP2D6 polymorphisms). If a breastfeeding mother has side-effects following codeine use, close monitoring should be exercised to identify any side-effects in the baby.

Nurses have an important role in mitigating the risks of medicines-related harm for particular groups and information from the genome can improve the safety and efficacy of treatment. CYP2D6 is a critical pharmacogene, responsible for the metabolism of around 20% of commonly prescribed medicines. It is highly polymorphic or subject to a number of variations which can be specific to certain populations. For example, a specific re-arrangement or hybridisation of the gene (CYP2D6-2D7) leading to a reduction in function is a phenomenon that appears widely in people of East Asian ethnicity. Variations in the function of CYP2D6, identified through genetic tests, that can accelerate or decelerate the production of morphine, leading to adverse effects from high plasma levels or sub-therapeutic plasma concentrations of drug which affect pain management, are seen more frequently in these groups (Taylor et al., 2020).

Tamoxifen

In the oncology setting, interactions between some cancer drugs and germline DNA can be anticipated in some patients and understanding variations in phenotype can help to predict and prevent harm from these treatments.

🔍 Case study

Michelle is 46 and has been diagnosed with oestrogen-receptor-positive breast cancer. As oestrogen can promote the growth and proliferation of cancer cells, her prescribing clinician is considering whether the selective oestrogen-receptor modulator, tamoxifen, would be an appropriate drug for Michelle. This drug inhibits the action of oestrogen upon cancer cell receptors.

Tamoxifen is a pro-drug, and the formation of its active metabolite endoxifen is mediated by the CYP2D6 enzyme. Michelle has an inherited CYP2D6 polymorphism that causes poor metabolism of drugs metabolised by CYP2D6. Michelle's dad also had this trait. For patients with the CYP2D6 poor metaboliser phenotype, increasing the standard dose by two or three times can achieve plasma concentrations of drug similar to those of normal metabolisers (de Dueñas et al., 2014).

Her prescriber discusses Michelle's options with her and decides to increase the starting dose of tamoxifen and to monitor the medication effects. Michelle responds well to the tamoxifen at the increased dose.

DPD deficiency

Fluoropyrimidine chemotherapy forms part of the essential treatment for some colorectal cancers. These drugs are precursors to active fluorouracil metabolites. Following their pharmacodynamic effects, the fluorouracil metabolites are rendered inactive for clearance by the liver enzyme dihydropyrimidine dehydrogenase or DPD (sometimes called DPYD). Inherited variants in the DPD gene can result in some level of DPD deficiency. If the deficiency is significant, treatment with this type of chemotherapy can lead rapidly to a life-threatening fluorouracil toxicity which could impact recovery and delay further treatment.

Testing for genomic variations which affect DPD levels is well established in cancer care. In those for whom treatment with these drugs is indicated, a blood test is taken to screen for the genetic variants that lead to DPD deficiency (Allen, 2021). A combined pharmacogenomic test for four variants which can predict up to 30% of severe 5-fluorouracil toxicities was commissioned by NHS England in 2020 and can now be carried out in any of the seven genomic laboratory hubs in the UK. When implementing the DPD deficiency test, NHS England commissioned concurrent work on ensuring equity of access to the tests for all (Sanghvi et al., 2023).

Q Case study

Paolo is 49 and has metastatic colorectal cancer. His oncologist, Clara, has recommended oral therapy with capecitabine. Capecitabine is metabolised to 5-fluorouracil. 5-fluorouracil is a substrate for DPD, and DPD testing is recommended prior to starting capecitabine to identify people at increased risk of drug toxicity. Paolo is tested for DPD deficiency before starting capecitabine. Results show that he has a heterozygous c.1905+ 1G>A (IVS14+1G>A) deficiency causing partial DPD deficiency (50% activity).

Clara looks at the UK Systemic Anti-cancer Therapy Board recommendations (Health Education England, 2023A) for recommendations on adjusting prescriptions in line with specific genotypes and discusses her findings with Paolo. They reach a shared decision to reduce the starting dose by one half to counterbalance the enzyme deficiency. If Paolo tolerates this dose, then it can be titrated up to 75% of the normal recommended starting dose. Appointments are scheduled with a specialist nurse check for serious adverse reaction such as myelosuppression and diarrhoea (Royal College of Physicians and British Pharmacological Society, 2022).

Reactive pharmacogenomic strategies such as this may be used in the context of a specific clinical situation, when a patient requires a specific drug to treat a specific condition. However, more pre-emptive pharmacogenomic testing of broad gene panels instead of single genes can be used to determine a pharmacogenomic profile for a patient. Individual profiles can be stored for future use across the lifespan. Although this is the direction of progress, systems have yet to be implemented to ensure that health care practitioners can access pharmacogenomic data at the point of prescribing (McDermott and Newman, 2023). In the UK, service improvements can be implemented nationally within the NHS, in contrast to the US, which hosts multiple county and state and other small private health organisations. This means that large-scale change is possible, but empirically, the NHS already struggles with shared access to patient record systems and fragmented care (Shepherd, 2016). Defined care pathways must be established with process guidelines for health care practitioners included in local policy and a clear governance structure.

Personalised medicine

Known drug–gene pair testing can underpin personalised medicine and as the evidence base grows, more pre-treatment pharmacogenomic tests are becoming integrated into practice settings (Clark, 2020). Pharmacogenomic testing can guide precision dosing, for example with drugs such as warfarin, to avoid adverse drug reactions, improve the impact of therapies and improve patient experience (Clark, 2020).

Nurses in many specialties may be required to clarify for patients what pharmacogenomic testing involves and why it may be relevant to their care. This knowledge will support patients to make informed choices about testing and subsequent treatment options. Patient pharmacogenomic education should take into account ethnic and cultural differences and preferences (Hicks et al., 2021). In some areas, following adequate training, nurses can obtain consent and order pharmacogenomic tests from laboratory hubs or conduct point of care tests. They can interpret and inform patients of their results and explain how test results will be used to plan safer treatment at the present time and in the future (Yousseff et al., 2020).

If a suspected polymorphism may affect an individual's response to more than one drug, for example, CYP2D6 variations can affect responses to SSRIs and to analgesia, single gene tests necessitate requesting only the information relevant to the prescribed medication (Haidar et al., 2022). Single-gene tests are less efficient than multi-gene panels but can achieve quicker results and remain cost effective in terms of avoiding medicines-related harm (Royal College of Physicians and British Pharmacological Society, 2022). Pharmacogenomic panel tests can be requested as drug or disease specific, for example tests can be requested to identify genetic variants relevant in the treatment of specific cancers. Tests can also be ordered to look for all pharmacogenes known to alter medication response. This type of test can provide many benefits in terms of treatment outcomes but also has some limitations. In addition to useful information, panel tests may include uncertain results which may present challenges for interpretation or use in informing prescribing decisions (Haidar et al., 2022).

All currently available gene targeted tests and pharmacogenomic gene panel tests are listed in the National Genomic Test Directory (NGTD). The NGTD contains sub-directories of tests to identify genetic and genomic diseases but also directories of the pharmacogenomic tests available for specific genes paired with commonly prescribed medications and for cancer drugs. It is important that nurses check the NGTD prior to discussing tests with patients in order to manage their expectations. In addition to the specific tests which are funded and available, the directory lists patient eligibility criteria and clinical actionability within the NHS technology, which helps to ensure national equity of access to pharmacogenomic testing (Royal College of Physicians and British Pharmacological Society, 2022).

There is a working group that assesses feasibility requests for pharmacogenomic tests to be added to the National Genomic Test Directory to ensure that patient needs are met across the UK. Tests may be added when there is robust evidence of a drug–gene association, evidence that clinical action can be taken if a variant is identified and evidence that acting on test results has the potential to improve outcomes. Tests should also be cost-effective, there must be no operational barriers within laboratory hubs and clinical guidance must be available to support the application of test results to prescribing (Sanghvi et al., 2023).

Reactive pharmacogenomic testing helps prescribers to decide whether the chosen treatment will be safe and effective, however, in these instances, results are not immediately available. Pre-emptive testing can be more efficient, where possible, so that relevant information is available at the point of prescribing to prompt a change in drug choice and to avoid the risk of medicines-related harm whilst waiting for results. The Preemptive Pharmacogenomic testing for pharmacogenes of Adverse drug Reactions (PREPARE) study was implemented to assess the cost-effectiveness of a pre-emptive panel-based approach to pharmacogenomic testing. Research showed a reduction in drug–genotype associated adverse drug reactions. Recommendations included a decrease in dose and careful monitoring for most drugs, and additional benefits to study participants included a reduction in other dose-related side effects and in side effects without a causal relationship to genes (van der Wouden et al., 2020).

Point of care pharmacogenetic testing

Frustration with the long turnaround time for many pharmacogenomic tests has expedited the development of point of care tests for use in the acute setting. Point of care pharmacogenomic testing is reactive testing at the point of prescribing, using a single-gene test for which immediate results can inform clinical decisions. This works well to improve prescribing for conditions where pharmacogenomic information enhances existing care pathways for example, phenotype-guided prescribing of clopidogrel following acute stroke (McDermott, 2023). The test is often as simple as obtaining a small sample, for example from a buccal swab, in a pre-mixed tube and putting the sample into a genotyping device. Results can take less than 1 hour and help to determine a safe and effective choice of drug and dose (Cheek, 2017).

Gentamicin

Individuals with variants in the RNR1 gene are pre-disposed to a risk of sensorineural hearing loss following the use of amino glycoside antibiotics such as gentamicin (Royal College of Physicians and British Pharmacological Society, 2022). The most common variant is m.1555A>G, present in approximately 1 in 500 people. One in 500 babies carry this genetic polymorphism and the risk of gentamicin-induced hearing loss is greater in infants owing to the immaturity and susceptibility to damage of the hair cells in the inner ear (Brown et al., 2024). Neonates admitted to the neonatal intensive care unit are usually given gentamicin within 60 minutes of admission to protect them from infection. The Manchester Pharmacogenetics to Avoid Loss of Hearing trial has directly contributed to new NICE (2023) early value assessment guidance (HTE6) to avoid ototoxicity from gentamicin use in newborns with the RNR1 variant (McDermott et al., 2021).

Following a successful pilot, a new point of care buccal swab has been introduced in practice which SCBU nurses can perform at the bedside. The test, which takes 26 minutes, can determine whether individual babies are at risk and could protect 180 babies in England each year from permanent hearing loss. Nurses are in a key position to implement genotyping in mainstream settings such as this. Exploring the views and utilising the knowledge and experience of nurses involved in implementing the point of care test was essential for its successful integration into existing care pathways. Training and support was required to build confidence but when surveyed, neonatal nurses reported that the test was valuable and being able to perform the test and to protect infants' hearing aligned with their values as nurses and helped them to fulfil their duty of care to babies and parents (Brown et al., 2024).

> ### 📖 Learning activity
>
> Design a parent/carer information leaflet to support obtaining consent for a new-born to receive a buccal swab in SCBU. The DNA sample will be used to test for a possible genetic variation which increases their susceptibility of ototoxicity following the use of gentamicin.
>
> (This learning activity is linked to NHS England (2023) genomic nursing competencies 2, 3 and 5.)

Barriers to the implementation of pharmacogenomics

While many health care practitioners can perceive the associated benefits of tests for patients there are some challenges to integrating pharmacogenomics into health services. High costs can be prohibitive to accessing available tests outside of specialist care settings such as oncology (Royal College of Physicians and British Pharmacological Society, 2022). Moreover, as a relatively new area, a lack of pharmacogenomics experience among health care professionals means that little empirical evidence exists for consultation. Additional research is required to understand drug-gene reactions and organisational care pathways and electronic systems must be updated, so prescribers can access information when needed (Royal College of Physicians and British Pharmacological Society, 2022). Healthcare practitioners will require adequate training to be able to interpret test results accurately from complex reporting terminology and apply this information to prescribing decisions (Rahma et al., 2020; McDermott and Newman, 2023). However, training needs for health care professionals have been a consistent barrier to the integration of genetic information into patient care (Hicks et al., 2021).

The CPIC has made efforts to standardise allele and phenotype terms, for example 'low function' or 'low activity' and to maintain consistent nomenclature to improve understanding and avoid confusion between settings (Caudle et al., 2017). Nevertheless, effective pharmacogenomic testing relies upon prescribers remembering that there is a drug-gene implication when prescribing certain drugs and having sufficient knowledge to modify treatment appropriately based on results. To support prescribers with this, active clinical decision support can be provided via pharmacogenomic alerts on e-prescribing systems (Haidar et al., 2022), although in oncology practice, frequent alerts for interactions between fluoropyrimidines and DPYD deficiency can cause alert fatigue resulting in reduced levels of acknowledgement and appropriate action (Hicks et al., 2021).

Owing to a lack of pharmacogenomics education, there has been an increased incidence of litigation related to the failure of health care practitioners to inform patients of potential medicines-related harms of which they were not themselves aware (Relling and Evans, 2015). Nurses prescribing and administering medications as part of their roles are accountable for accessing safety information and for following warnings implemented by medicines and health care products regulatory agencies (Royal College of Physicians and British Pharmacological Society, 2022).

In order to realise the advantages pharmacogenomic tests offer, patient results should be easy for prescribers to access when required, although organisational data management processes must take into account privacy and confidentiality regulations. The results from pharmacogenomic tests could be used to discriminate against individuals and could affect their health insurance (Rahma et al., 2020). Other new and potentially problematic ethical issues associated with pharmacogenomic tests include the disclosure of incidental findings. When reporting the results of pharmacogenomic tests, nurses must note which results the patient has consented to receive and only the information from testing which is relevant to maintain patient safety regarding the specific medicines to be prescribed. Practitioners taking consent must bear this in mind and record patient preferences beforehand to avoid subsequent problems.

Pharmacogenomics and ethnicity

Culturally competent care is discussed in Chapters 3 and 6. It is also important to highlight the effects that ethnicity may have on medicines safety and efficacy and the value of pharmacogenomic information when caring for different groups. A much greater frequency of pharmacogenetic variants occurs in non-European populations, including rarer variations not captured by the current recording system (McInnes et al., 2021).

The British-South Asian population has a high number of intermediate or poor CYP2C19 metabolisers. This creates implications for drugs such as clopidogrel, which must be metabolised by CYP2C19 into their active form to reach optimal clinical efficacy. Poor metabolisers who receive clopidogrel following an acute myocardial infarction are more likely to have a repeat occurrence. Careful monitoring of this medication is recommended, and tests are being developed to identify other genetic polymorphisms contributing to reduced drug efficacy (Magavern et al., 2023).

Carbamazepine

Genetic polymorphisms or common variations in genes between individuals and populations can affect individual responses to certain drugs. This includes a pre-disposition to or increased risk of individual reactions such as drug allergy or sensitivity, leading to type B adverse drug reactions (Coulson, 2021). An individual's genetics can predispose them to allergic reactions and the presence of the HLA-B*1502 allele is highly associated with carbamazepine-induced Stevens–Johnson syndrome and toxic epidermal necrolysis. This association has been found mostly in those of Han Chinese origin and the BNF recommends pre-treatment screening for this variation in individuals of Han Chinese or Thai origin.

Prescribers are advised to order pre-treatment screening 'where possible' but the test may not be available in all areas as an equitable national pharmacogenomics service has yet to be established as a core part of the NHS (Royal College of Physicians and British Pharmacological Society, 2022). Other anti-seizure medications such as oxcarbazepine and phenytoin have also been linked to Stevens–Johnson syndrome, but the risk factors are not as well defined as for carbamazepine (Relling and Evans, 2015). Pharmacogenomic information such as this can help improve patient outcomes but also reduce cost to the NHS from ADRs which are estimated to total over £2.2 billion annually, including the cost of preventable hospital admissions (McDermott and Newman, 2023).

⟨⟩ Skills focus – identifying Stevens–Johnson syndrome

Pharmacovigilance is an important skill that helps nurses to prevent or reduce medicines related harm. When Stevens–Johnson syndrome is suspected the drug must be discontinued and immediate medical help sought. Stevens–Johnson syndrome can be recognised by the following signs and symptoms:

- flu-like malaise and fever;
- ocular, oral and genital lesions, spots or blisters;
- in the acute phase, patients are at risk of septicaemia and renal failure;
- the condition can develop to include oesophageal erosion and stricture and pulmonary and hepatic involvement (Lerch et al., 2018).

Anti-thrombotic agents

Across health care settings, many nurses without specialised training will be responsible for caring for patients with pharmacogenomic considerations and for educating them about the potential effects and the importance of adherence or taking their medicines exactly as prescribed. It is estimated that up to 30 genes interact with warfarin, a commonly prescribed anticoagulant (Munroe and Loerzal, 2016). Warfarin has a narrow therapeutic range, so it is important to avoid plasma concentrations which are too high or too low, which can be harmful or lead to an ineffective response. Fluctuations in plasma levels can be caused by alterations in metabolism and cause challenges in maintaining an international normalised ratio within the normal range. Data from point of care tests on polymorphisms which affect drug efficacy contribute to dose decisions and improved anti-coagulation control, increasing the safety and effectiveness of prescribing (Jorgensen et al., 2019).

Allopurinol

There is an association between HLA-B*5801 and the increased risk of Stevens–Johnson syndrome for some patients when taking allopurinol for gout (Chair et al., 2019).

Mavacamten

Individuals with loss of function in two CYP2C19 alleles will metabolise mavacamten poorly. This drug is used to treat hypertrophic cardiomyopathy and increased exposure from high plasma levels of drug can lead to an increased clinical effect, causing systolic dysfunction (Health Education England, 2023B).

Collecting information

Nurses should report severe or unusual drug reactions to the Medicines and Healthcare Products Regulatory Agency (MHRA) via the yellow card system.

Yellow card reporting for ADRs

- ADRs can be reported by any patient, carer or health care professional.
- Any ADR can be reported through the MHRA yellow card website.
- It is particularly important to report ADRs which may add to the evidence base to prevent future ADRs. This includes severe ADRs and ADRs experienced by pregnant women and children for whom there are fewer sources of research owing to ethical concerns which place restrictions on research trials.
- The MHRA is also starting to collect data on drug–gene pairs to help prevent ADRs related to specific drugs in individuals with genetic polymorphisms (MHRA, 2024).

The yellow card Biobank, set up by the MHRA in 2023, is a large biomedical database that contains detailed genetic and health information from more than half a million people living in the UK.

The Biobank houses genetic information from people who have had drug reactions in order to highlight common pairs of reactions and traits. Data collection enables researchers and health care practitioners to better understand how different phenotypes affect responses to medications and to predict and prevent future adverse reactions to medicines. At this time nurses can complete report cards for suspected pharmacogenomic adverse reactions following allopurinol and excessive bleeding following the use of DOACs such as rivaroxaban, dabigatran, apixaban and edoxaban (MHRA, 2024).

Building the evidence base is vital for the compilation of new safety guidelines and the integration of pharmacogenomics into mainstream health care. Pharmacogenomic data can also be used to support medicines optimisation. Various consortia have been established globally to collect, store and share data which facilitates the advancement of personalised medicine and medicines safety. The Ubiquitous Pharmacogenomics Consortium investigates the impact of pharmacogenomics on patient outcomes and any impact on health care costs (Hetland et al., 2024). The Pharmacogene Variation Consortium (PharmVar, https://www.pharmvar.org/) is a US repository for drug–gene pairing information to facilitate research on clinically actionable pharmacogenetic variations. PharmVar catalogues high impact pharmacogenetic variations using the 'star alleles' nomenclature system (McInnes et al., 2021).

Some other organisations publish widely recognised, evidence-based pharmacogenomic-prescribing recommendations, for example the Dutch Pharmacokinetics Working Group (DPWG) established in the Netherlands in 2005, and the Clinical Pharmacogenetics Implementation Consortium (CPIC) established in the US in 2009

(Bank et al., 2017). The DPWG and the CPIC systematically review pharmacogenetic literature from individual case studies through to randomised controlled trials, to produce standardised guidelines on pharmacogenomic variants, their effects, test results and drug dosage (McDermott and Newman, 2023).

UK drug labelling has changed in line with pharmacogenomic discovery and brief guidance is now provided by manufacturers on pharmacogenomic guided prescribing for some products. For example, pharmaceutical companies which make carbamazepine recommend within its summary of product characteristics that individuals of Han Chinese or Thai origin have a genetic test prior to treatment where possible to avoid preventable reactions (Royal College of Physicians and British Pharmacological Society, 2022). This practice has also been adopted by the European Medicines Agency with new drugs including information about genetic biomarkers (Clark, 2020). In the US, the FDA (2024) provide a list of current medicines prescribed nationally with pharmacogenomic information within drug labelling.

⚛ UK Biobank

- UK Biobank is a large biomedical database that enables new discoveries to improve public health.
- Patients who are recruited and wish to contribute to this research must visit an assessment centre to provide data about themselves and biological samples such as blood and urine.
- They must provide informed consent to contribute data to the Biobank: https://www.ukbiobank.ac.uk/media/05ldg1ez/consent-form-uk-biobank.pdf
- Anonymised genetic data can be accessed by researchers globally, upon application, to improve understanding of genetic conditions.
- The UK Biobank made a significant contribution to managing the COVID-19 pandemic through antibody testing and data sharing (UK Biobank, 2023).

Clinical guidance

Decision support, for example within electronic prescribing systems or from pharmacists, can help nurse prescribers use information from individual genetic profiles to prescribe safely by helping them to balance the likelihood of achieving a therapeutic effect from a drug with the risk of harm. Alongside information obtained through pharmacogenomic testing, professional guidance helps nurses to make shared decisions with patients regarding their options and to gain informed consent for treatment. Nurses can also help to support patient adherence to medication by discussing possible side effects and how they might be managed prior to treatment (NICE, 2015).

Giving information effectively and implementing strategies to prevent avoidable harm assists nurses administering and monitoring the effects of medication to maintain patient safety. Nurses can promote pharmacogenomic testing when indicated to help prevent genetically pre-determined drug reactions or reduced clinical efficacy when using some drugs. However, pre-test counselling regarding pharmacogenomic testing options and possible outcomes, including possible restrictions on treatment choices to avoid harm requires the development of relevant knowledge and the ability to access current evidence (Royal College of Physicians and British Pharmacological Society, 2022).

Evidence to support the safety benefits of pharmacogenomic tests for patients in relation to their medicines regimes is increasing in volume but it can be challenging to translate scientific research in this area into clinical practice. Past barriers to the effective clinical integration of pharmacogenomics have included a paucity of evidence-based practice guidelines for the management of known drug–gene pairs (Relling and Evans, 2015). However, an increased volume of research is taking place, and some databases continue to collect and refine pharmacogenomic data. Table 7.1, at the end of this chapter, contains a summary of some known drug-gene pairs and options for clinical management.

PharmGKB (https://www.pharmgkb.org/) is a pharmacogenomics 'knowledge base' developed by Stanford University with funding from the NIH, which combines information and guidance from the CPIC, the DPWG and the FDA. Prescribers can search for information by gene or by variant. This resource also lists commonly prescribed medicines for which pharmacogenomic prescribing recommendations are available and gives individualised pharmacogenomic recommendations for adults and children. It is a publicly available tool that encompasses comprehensive clinical data on both the impact of genetic variation on treatment response and potentially actionable associated drug-gene pairs for health care practitioners.

Adequate preparation of the nursing workforce is required to facilitate access to relevant information to underpin pharmacogenomics related care. The nursing community will require focused education regarding the interpretation of and actionability of findings related to drug–gene pairs to benefit their patients. This is beginning to happen in some areas, for example large oncology centres but a lack of empirical research into how the nursing role has adapted to include pharmacogenomic related care has not permitted much insight into other specific measures required for meaningful forward momentum (Hetland et al., 2024).

🩺 Skills focus – identify pharmacogenomic risk by:

- asking the right questions when taking a medicines history, including questions related to drug reactions or therapeutic failure in the past;
- asking patients about drug reactions or therapeutic failure in family members (Cheek, 2017);
- identifying when individuals are from high-risk ethnic populations; and
- reading the safety information given in BNF drug monographs.

Abacavir

Antiretroviral therapies such as abacavir, which may be prescribed to inhibit HIV replication, are a cornerstone of HIV management. However, abacavir is contraindicated in patients who have the HLA-B*5701 allele, which can increase their risk of hypersensitivity to this drug. HLA stands for Human Leucocyte Antigen and hypersensitivity

Table 7.1 Common drug–gene pairs

Genetic polymorphism	Drug or drug group implicated	Effect (varies according to patient phenotype)	Clinical guidance
NUDT15 TPMT	Thiopurines	Slow drug metabolism and/or reduced tolerance (Relling et al., 2018). Risk of severe leucopoenia (van der Wouden et al., 2020)	Pre-treatment testing (Haidar et al., 2022, Relling et al., 2018). Genotype based dose reduction in line with CPIC guidance (Bank et al., 2017)
CYP2C9 and VKORC1	Anti-coagulants such as warfarin	Reduced drug efficacy and risk of internal or external bleeding (Clark, 2020)	Decrease loading dose (Bank et al., 2017). Genotype guided warfarin therapy or consider direct oral anti-coagulant therapy (Sanghvi et al., 2023)
CYP2C19*2	Anti-platelet agents such as clopidogrel	Reduced function and lower concentrations of active metabolite impacts clinical efficacy (Magavern et al., 2023)	Pre-treatment point of care screening in development. Monitor medication effects
CYP2D6	Codeine	Slow or fast metabolism (depending on phenotype). Side effects or sub-optimal therapy	Pre-treatment testing if high risk. Monitor medication effects. Consider alternative therapy when necessary (Relling and Evans, 2015)
CYP3A5	Tacrolimus	Difficulty achieving therapeutic plasma concentration	Monitor medication effects (Sanghvi et al., 2023). Adjust dose as appropriate (Relling and Evans, 2015)
HLA-B*1502 HLA-A*3101	Carbamazepine	Increased risk of Stevens–Johnson syndrome and toxic epidermal necrolysis. Increased risk of cutaneous adverse reactions	Pre-treatment testing for Han Chinese or Thai patients (Joint Formulary Committee, 2024). Or use alternative antiepileptics (Sanghvi et al., 2023). In individuals of European or Japanese origin consider use only if potential benefit outweighs risk (Joint Formulary Committee, 2024)
CYP2C9	Phenytoin	Phenytoin induced toxicities	25% reduction in starting dose, monitor and adjust maintenance doses in line with response (Caudle et al., 2017)

Gene	Drug	Effect	Action
CYP2D6 CYP2C19	SSRI (selective serotonin reuptake inhibitors) or anti-depressants such as fluoxetine, paroxetine, citalopram and sertraline	Fast metabolism, poor response	Consider an alternative drug (Caudle et al., 2017)
CYP2D6 CYP2C19	Tricyclic anti-depressants such as amitriptyline and clomipramine	Slow or fast metabolism. Side effects or sub-optimal therapy	Consider an alternative drug (Bank et al., 2017)
HLA-B*5701	Abacavir	Hypersensitivity	Pre-treatment testing where available. Or monitor for signs of a reaction within first 6 weeks or hypersensitivity at any time during use (Cheek, 2017)
SLCO1B1	Statins	Statin associated myopathy	Consider genotype in conjunction with other risk factors and review current CPIC and/or DPWG guidelines prior to adjusting any prescription (Health Education England, 2023C)
CYP2C19	Mavacamten	Poor metabolism leading to systolic dysfunction	Pre-treatment prospective screening and reduction starting dose if poor metaboliser genotype identified (Health Education England, 2023B)
NFKB1 SLC39A8	Short acting bronchodilators such as albuterol	Reduced response, poor asthmatic control	Prescribe in line with individual response
CYP2C19	PPIs such as omeprazole	*Improves* efficacy (van der Wouden et al., 2022)	
CYP2C9	Non-steroidal anti-inflammatory drugs such as ibuprofen	Gastrointestinal, renal and cardiovascular events (McDermott and Newman, 2023)	Monitor treatment effects and discontinue drug or adjust prescription as appropriate

(Continued)

Table 7.1 Common drug–gene pairs *(continued)*

Genetic polymorphism	Drug or drug group implicated	Effect (varies according to patient phenotype)	Clinical guidance
DPYD (or DPD)	Fluoropyrimidines such as capecitabine	Reduced or absent metabolism of toxic metabolite (5-fluorouracil)	Consider an alternative drug (Bank et al., 2017)
HLA-B	Allopurinol	Severe cutaneous adverse reaction such as Stevens–Johnson syndrome (McDermott and Newman, 2023)	Monitor treatment effects and discontinue drug if cutaneous reaction
m.1555A>G	Aminoglycoside antibiotics such as gentamicin	Vestibulotoxicity and aminoglycoside induced sensorineural hearing loss	Pre-treatment screening (a mitochondrial RNR1 test) and genotype guided antibiotic prescription (Sanghvi et al., 2023)

CPIC, Clinical Pharmacogenetics Implementation Consortium.

reactions may be identified by flu-like symptoms in conjunction with gastro-intestinal symptoms, usually experienced within the first 6 weeks of treatment (Cheek et al., 2017; Youssef et al., 2020). A reaction to a specific treatment can have serious implications for HIV therapy as it can often be challenging to find drugs with tolerable side effects. Patients may have trouble getting used to some treatments and the impact on their lifestyle can reduce the likelihood of medication adherence. Pharmacogenomic testing can eliminate the trial-and-error approach to prescribing (van der Wouden et al., 2020) and testing for allelic variation reduces the risk of hypersensitivity reactions to abacavir and is therefore cost effective (Royal College of Physicians and British Pharmacological Society, 2022).

> ### ☼ Reflection point – HIV treatment, patient experience and nursing care:
>
> - imagine you have HIV;
> - consider how it might feel to become hypersensitive to a medication which has so far worked well to control your symptoms;
> - outline the areas of your life upon which this could impact; and
> - list the questions you might have for an HIV specialist nurse.

Thiopurines

Thiopurine methyltransferase (TPMT) variant alleles are associated with decreased enzyme activity and increased exposure to drugs such as azathioprine, mercaptopurine and thioguanine which are prescribed for the treatment of non-malignant immunological disorders. Because genetically pre-determined TPMT levels affect the metabolism of these drugs, obtaining accurate information through pre-treatment testing can help prescribers to adjust doses as appropriate and to improve outcomes from treatment. Loss of function alleles in the NUDT15 genes are common in Asian and Hispanic ethnicities and can affect clearance of these drugs or their active metabolites (mercaptopurine is a metabolite of azathioprine) (Relling et al., 2019).

Pharmacogenomic testing in children

Evidence has shown that pharmacogenomic testing can improve medicines safety in paediatric medicine in the same way as for adults. Specific examples include TPMT testing prior to the use of thiopurines to treat paediatric leukaemia, which has been shown to improve efficacy and help avoid harmful ADRs (Botkin et al., 2015).

Childhood asthma is very common and has strong genetic associations. Varied response to different types of treatment for asthma has long been a challenge and can result in poor control. Some populations, for example those of Japanese descent are more at risk of treatment failure owing to genetic variation (Gupta and Awasthi, 2010). Albuterol is a first-line treatment that can be used to relieve respiratory distress in children with asthma. Beta2 adrenergic receptor gene variants can affect response to this drug and identification of variants can improve outcomes through tailoring the drug to the individual response (Jaekel, 2012). It is reported that albuterol is the most commonly prescribed inhaler and sometimes the only choice available within poorer communities. However, albuterol and some other inhaled medicines do not work as well in children. Owing to a recently discovered genetic variation, research has also shown that inhalers do not work as well in Puerto-Rican and

African American children in the US, who represent the paediatric population with the largest global prevalence of asthma (Weiler, 2018).

Mental health

Individuals who are fast metabolisers of some antidepressant medications can achieve only subtherapeutic plasma concentrations and receive little therapeutic benefit from these drugs. This can be distressing for patients with unremitting symptoms. Pharmacogenomic testing can help to identify and avoid antidepressants that may be inappropriate owing to genetic polymorphisms (Yousseff et al., 2020). People with major depressive disorder are more likely to achieve symptom remission when receiving pharmacogenomic-guided treatment (Bousman et al., 2019).

Recent pharmacogenomic research

- The US trial for Implementation of Point-of-Care Pharmacogenomic Decision Support in Perioperative Care research has been implemented to determine whether pre-emptive pharmacogenomic genotyping can support peri-operative medicines safety (Truong et al., 2019).
- The Pharmacogenetics Roll Out – Gauging Response to Service project, led by the Northwest Genomic Medicine Service Alliance, aims to establish the feasibility of delivering pharmacogenomic gene panel test results for patients in primary care (NHS, 2023). In some UK regions, nurses and clinicians have been obtaining consent to test for polymorphisms before prescribing 'trigger meds' such as statins, some anti-depressants (tricyclic and SSRIs) or proton pump inhibitors. The aim of this research is to develop a system to translate pharmacogenomic test results into prescribing advice for GPs and around one-quarter of the 400 participants in the trial have had their prescriptions changed as a result of their genomic test results (Willis, 2024). There is a YouTube video (https://www.youtube.com/watch?v=FjWpZiy8zS0) for patients explaining the benefits of testing and of collecting data for research
- Cohn et al. (2021) combined point of care pharmacogenomic testing and pre-emptive pharmacogenomic screening in a Canadian children's hospital to inform prescribing for children with heart conditions. The children enrolled in this study had experienced low therapeutic benefit from previous treatments and clinicians found that having genomic data available permitted the use of a greater range of drugs and guided dosing decisions to provide individualised and improved care.

Summary

Pharmacogenomics is concerned with predicting individual responses to medicine to prevent harm. Pharmacogenomic tests can highlight polymorphisms which may affect a person's response to a specific drug. Information from tests can be kept in a person's health records to ensure future efficacy in prescribing and prevent harm. Nurses should be aware of how pharmacogenomic information contributes to the safer prescribing and administration of medicines.

Learn more

- The Health Education England Genomics Education Programme knowledge hub is comprehensive and informative and includes prescribing support, including useful tables on drug–gene pairs: https://www.genomicseducation.hee.nhs.uk/genotes/knowledge-hub/introduction-to-pharmacogenomics/

■ GeNotes, produced as part of the Health Education England Genomics Education Programme (2023), outline a number of different clinical scenarios where a presenting patient might require pre-treatment testing before being prescribed a particular drug, to support clinical decision making: https://www.genomicseducation.hee.nhs.uk/genotes/pharmacogenomics/

■ The Medicines Learning Portal is a clinical problem-solving resource designed for pharmacists. This resource contains links to many sources of useful information for all health care professionals: https://www.medicineslearningportal.org/2024/03/pharmacogenomics-making-decisions-about.html

Resources for patients

■ This short video produced by the University of Utah explains the principles of pharmacogenomics and how they underpin safe prescribing choices: https://learn.genetics.utah.edu/content/precision/example

---

(?) **Test yourself – pharmacogenomics quiz**

1. Explain what pharmacogenomics means.
2. Explain how genetic variation to pharmacokinetic processing can create a risk of medicines related harm.
3. Give an example of a drug or patient group where genetic polymorphisms can increase the risk of an allergic or sensitivity-type reaction.
4. List six drugs or drug groups implicated in pharmacogenomic risk.

Quiz answers

1. Pharmacogenomics is a branch of pharmacology related to predicting individual responses to medicines determined by genetic variation in order to improve medicines safety.
2. A genetic liver enzyme deficiency can reduce the metabolism of drugs metabolised by that enzyme. This is usually a CYP450 enzyme. Reduced metabolism increases plasma concentration of drug, which may lead to increased clinical effect or effects at unintended sites.
3. Some genetic polymorphisms can pre-dispose individuals to a higher risk of adverse drug reactions. These include carbamazepine which can increase the risk of Stevens–Johnson syndrome in those who have a variation in the HLA-B*1502 gene. Groups at risk include those of Han Chinese or Thai origin.
4. Anticoagulants, anti-platelets, codeine, thiopurines, fluoropyrimidines, carbamazepine, abacavir, albuterol, statins, anti-depressants, tacrolimus, phenytoin, selective serotonin reuptake inhibitors (SSRIs), tricyclic anti-depressants, mavacamten, short acting bronchodilators, proton pump inhibitors, non-steroidal anti-inflammatory drugs (NSAIDs), allopurinol, and aminoglycoside antibiotics.

References

Allen, D., 2021. Cancer nursing and genomics. *Cancer Nursing Practice*, 20(2), pp.17–19.

Bank, P.C.D., Caudle, K.E., Swen, J.J., Gammal, R.S., Whirl-Carrillo, M., Klein, T.E., Relling, M.V. and Guchelaar, H.J., 2017. Comparison of the guidelines of the clinical pharmacogenetics implementation consortium and the Dutch pharmacogenetics working group. *Clinical Pharmacology & Therapeutics*, 103(4), pp.599–618.

Botkin, J.R., Belmont, J.W., Berg, J.S., Berkman, B.E., Bombard, Y., Holm, I.A., Levy, H.P., Ormond, K.E., Saal, H.M., Spinner, N.B. and Wilfond, B.S., 2015. Points to consider: ethical, legal, and psychosocial implications of genetic testing in children and adolescents. *The American Journal of Human Genetics*, 97(1), pp.6–21.

Bousman CA, Arandjelovic K, Mancuso SG et al., 2019. Pharmacogenetic tests and depressive symptom remission: a meta-analysis of randomized controlled trials. *Pharmacogenomics*, 20(1), 37–47. Doi: 10.2217/pgs-2018-0142

Brown, G., Warrington, N., Ulph, F., Booth, N., Harvey, K., James, R., Tricker, K., Wilson, P., Newman, W., Mcdermott, J.H. and Stoddard, D., 2024. Exploring NICU nurses' views of a novel genetic point-of-care test identifying neonates at risk of antibiotic-induced ototoxicity: a qualitative study. *Journal of Advanced Nursing*, 80(8), pp.3359–3370.

Caudle, K.E., Dunnenberger, H.M., Freimuth, R.R., Peterson, J.F., Burlison, J.D., Whirl-Carrillo, M., Scott, S.A., Rehm, H.L., Williams, M.S., Klein, T.E. and Relling, M.V., 2017. Standardizing terms for clinical pharmacogenetic test results: consensus terms from the Clinical Pharmacogenetics Implementation Consortium (CPIC). *Genetics in Medicine*, 19(2), pp.215–223.

Chair, S.Y., Waye, M.M.Y., Calzone, K. and Chan, C.W.H., 2019. Genomics education in nursing in Hong Kong, Taiwan and mainland China. *International Nursing Review*, 66(4), pp.459–466.

Cheek, D.J., 2017. Pharmacogenomics: strategies for individualized *care. Nursing2020 Critical Care*, 12(1), pp.22–27.

Clark, T., 2020. *Genomic Innovation: Technologies for Personalised Medicine*. The AHSN network.

Cohn, I., Manshaei, R., Liston, E., Okello, J.B., Khan, R., Curtis, M.R., Krupski, A.J., Jobling, R.K., Kalbfleisch, K., Paton, T.A. and Reuter, M.S., 2021. Assessment of the implementation of pharmacogenomic testing in a pediatric tertiary care setting. *JAMA Network Open*, 4(5), pp.e2110446–e2110446.

Coulson, J., 2021. Understanding the pharmacology of the side effects of medicines for effective prevention of adverse drug reactions. *Nursing Standard (Royal College of Nursing (Great Britain): 1987)*, 37(3), pp.60–66.

Cox, F., Cannons, K., Lewis, S. et al., 2015. *Pain Knowledge and Skills Framework for the Nursing Team*. Royal College of Nursing: London.

de Dueñas, E.M., Aranda, E.O., Lopez-Barajas, I.B., Magdalena, T.F., Moya, F.B., García, L.M.C., Capilla, J.A.G., Ceres, M.Z., de Haro, T., Llorens, R.R. and Albiach, C.F., 2014. Adjusting the dose of tamoxifen in patients with early breast cancer and CYP2D6 poor metabolizer phenotype. *The Breast*, 23(4), pp.400–406.

FDA, 2024. Table of pharmacogenomic biomarkers in drug labeling. https://www.fda.gov/drugs/science-and-research-drugs/table-pharmacogenomic-biomarkers-drug-labeling (accessed 4 July 2024).

Gupta, S. and Awasthi, S., 2010. Pharmacogenomics of pediatric asthma. *Indian Journal of Human Genetics*, 16(3), p.111.

Haidar, C.E., Crews, K.R., Hoffman, J.M., Relling, M.V. and Caudle, K.E., 2022. Advancing pharmacogenomics from single-gene to pre-emptive testing. *Annual Review of Genomics and Human Genetics*, 23, pp.449–473.

Health Education England, 2023A. Ge Notes. https://www.genomicseducation.hee.nhs.uk/genotes/in-the-clinic/results-patient-with-known-dpyd-variants-requiring-fluoropyrimidine-based-chemotherapy/ (accessed 20 June 2024).

Health Education England, 2023B. Ge notes. https://www.genomicseducation.hee.nhs.uk/genotes/in-the-clinic/results-patient-with-hypertrophic-cardiomyopathy-with-known-cyp2c19-genotype-requiring-mavacamten/ (accessed 1 August 2024).

Health Education England, 2023C. Ge notes. https://www.genomicseducation.hee.nhs.uk/genotes/in-the-clinic/results-patient-with-known-slco1b1-genotype-requiring-statin-therapy/ (accessed 1 August 2024).

Hetland, L.H., Maguire, J., Debono, D. and Wright, H., 2024. Scholarly literature on nurses and pharmacogenomics: A scoping review. *Nurse Education Today*, 137, p.106153.

Hicks, J.K., Howard, R., Reisman, P., Adashek, J.J., Fields, K.K., Gray, J.E., McIver, B., McKee, K., O'Leary, M.F., Perkins, R.M. and Robinson, E., 2021. Integrating somatic and germline next-generation sequencing into routine clinical oncology practice. *JCO Precision Oncology*, 5, pp.884–895.

Jaekel, R.C.J., 2012. Nursing students' knowledge of genetics and genomics: an online module (Doctoral dissertation, Texas Woman's University).

Joint Formulary Committee, 2024. Carbamazepine. British National Formulary. https://bnf.nice.org.uk/drugs/carbamazepine/#cautions (accessed 19 May 2024).

Jorgensen, A.L., Prince, C., Fitzgerald, G., Hanson, A., Downing, J., Reynolds, J., Zhang, J.E., Alfirevic, A. and Pirmohamed, M., 2019. Implementation of genotype-guided dosing of warfarin with point-of-care genetic testing in three UK clinics: a matched cohort study. *BMC Medicine*, 17, pp.1–11.

Lea, D.H., Skirton, H., Read, C.Y. and Williams, J.K., 2011. Implications for educating the next generation of nurses on genetics and genomics in the 21st century. *Journal of Nursing Scholarship*, 43(1), pp.3–12.

Lerch, M., Mainetti, C., Terziroli Beretta-Piccoli, B. and Harr, T., 2018. Current perspectives on Stevens–Johnson syndrome and toxic epidermal necrolysis. *Clinical Reviews in Allergy & Immunology*, 54, pp.147–176.

Magavern, E.F., Jacobs, B., Warren, H., Finocchiaro, G., Finer, S., Genes & Health Research Team, van Heel, D.A., Smedley, D. and Caulfield, M.J., 2023. CYP2C19 Genotype prevalence and association with recurrent myocardial infarction in British–South Asians treated with clopidogrel. *JACC: Advances*, 2(7), p.100573.

McDermott, J.H. 2023. Point-of-care pharmacogenomic testing. https://www.genomicseducation.hee.nhs.uk/genotes/knowledge-hub/point-of-care-pharmacogenomic-testing/ (accessed 3 July 2024)

McDermott, J.H. and Newman, W., 2023. Introduction to pharmacogenetics. *Drug and Therapeutics Bulletin*, 61(11), pp.168–172.

McDermott, J.H., Mahood, R., Stoddard, D., Mahaveer, A., Turner, M.A., Corry, R., Garlick, J., Miele, G., Ainsworth, S., Kemp, L. and Bruce, I., 2021. Pharmacogenetics to avoid loss of hearing (PALOH) trial: a protocol for a prospective observational implementation trial. *BMJ Open*, 11(6), p.e044457.

McGavock, H., 2017. *How Drugs Work: Basic Pharmacology for Health Professionals*. CRC Press: Boca Raton, FL.

McInnes, G., Lavertu, A., Sangkuhl, K., Klein, T.E., Whirl-Carrillo, M. and Altman, R.B., 2021. Pharmacogenetics at scale: an analysis of the UK Biobank. *Clinical Pharmacology & Therapeutics*, 109(6), pp.1528–1537.

MHRA, 2014. Drug safety update codeine: very rare risk of side-effects in breastfed babies. https://www.gov.uk/drug-safety-update/codeine-very-rare-risk-of-side-effects-in-breastfed-babies

MHRA, 2024. Biobank. https://yellowcard.mhra.gov.uk/biobank (accessed 1 August 2024).

Munroe, T. and Loerzel, V., 2016. Assessing nursing students' knowledge of genomic concepts and readiness for use in practice. *Nurse Educator*, 41(2), pp.86–89.

NHS, 2023. North West GMSA spotlight: PROGRESS project. https://www.nw-gmsa.nhs.uk/about-us/our-projects/spotlight (accessed 4 July 2024).

NHS England, 2023. The 2023 genomic competency framework for UK nurses. https://www.genomicseducation.hee.nhs.uk/wp-content/uploads/2023/12/2023-Genomic-Competency-Framework-for-UK-Nurses.pdf

NHS England, 2024. NHS Genomics Networks of Excellence. https://pharmaceutical-journal. com/article/news/pharmacogenomics-and-medicines-optimisation-one-of-eight-nhs-genomic-networks-of-excellence (accessed 1 August 2024).

NICE, 2015. Medicines optimisation: the safe and effective use of medicines to enable the best possible outcomes. https://www.nice.org.uk/guidance/ng5

NICE, 2023. Genedrive MT-RNR1 ID Kit for detecting a genetic variant to guide antibiotic use and prevent hearing loss in babies: early value assessment. https://www.nice.org.uk/guidance/hte6

NICE, 2024A. News. https://www.nice.org.uk/news/articles/nice-launches-second-consultation-on-genetic-testing-to-guide-treatment-after-a-stroke (accessed 21 June 2024).

NICE, 2024B. CYP2C19 genotype testing to guide clopidogrel use after ischaemic stroke or transient ischaemic attack. https://www.nice.org.uk/guidance/dg59

Nursing and Midwifery Council, 2018. *Standards of Proficiency for Registered Nurses.* NMC: London.

Rahma, A.T., Elsheik, M., Ali, B.R., Elbarazi, I., Patrinos, G.P., Ahmed, L.A. and Al Maskari, F., 2020. Knowledge, attitudes, and perceived barriers toward genetic testing and pharmacogenomics among healthcare workers in the United Arab Emirates: a cross-sectional study. *Journal of Personalized Medicine*, 10(4), p.216.

Relling, M.V. and Evans, W.E., 2015. Pharmacogenomics in the clinic. *Nature*, 526(7573), pp.343–350.

Relling, M.V., Schwab, M., Whirl-Carrillo, M., Suarez-Kurtz, G., Pui, C.H., Stein, C.M., Moyer, A.M., Evans, W.E., Klein, T.E., Antillon-Klussmann, F.G. and Caudle, K.E., 2019. Clinical pharmacogenetics implementation consortium guideline for thiopurine dosing based on TPMT and NUDT 15 genotypes: 2018 update. *Clinical Pharmacology & Therapeutics*, 105(5), pp.1095–1105.

Royal College of Physicians and British Pharmacological Society joint working party, 2022. Personalised Prescribing: Using pharmacogenomics to improve outcomes. https://www.bps.ac.uk/getmedia/b43a3dca-1bbf-4bff-9379-20bef9349a8c/Personalised-prescribing-full-report.pdf.aspx

Royal Pharmaceutical Society, 2013. *Medicines Optimisation: Helping Patients to Make the Most of Medicines.* London: Royal Pharmaceutical Society. https://www.rpharms.com/Portals/0/RPS%20document%20library/Open%20access/Policy/helping-patients-make-the-most-of-their-medicines.pdf

Royal Pharmaceutical Society, 2019. *Professional Guidance on the Administration of Medicines in Healthcare Settings.* London: Royal Pharmaceutical Society. https://www.rpharms.com/Portals/0/RPS%20document%20library/Open%20access/Professional%20standards/SSHM%20and%20Admin/Admin%20of%20Meds%20prof%20guidance.pdf

Sanghvi, S., Ferner, R.E., Scourfield, A., Urquhart, R., Amin, S., Hingorani, A.D. and Sofat, R., 2023. How to assess pharmacogenomic tests for implementation in the NHS in England. *British Journal of Clinical Pharmacology*, 89(9), pp.2649–2657.

Shepherd, S., 2016. Coordinated care: a patient perspective on the impact of a fragmented system of care on experiences and outcomes, drawing on practical examples. *Future Healthcare Journal*, 3(2), pp.136–138.

Taylor, C., Crosby, I., Yip, V., Maguire, P., Pirmohamed, M. and Turner, R.M., 2020. A Review of the Important Role of CYP2D6 in Pharmacogenomics. *Genes*, 11(11), p.1295.

Truong, T.M., Apfelbaum, J., Shahul, S., Anitescu, M., Danahey, K., Knoebel, R.W., Liebovitz, D., Karrison, T., van Wijk, X.M., Yeo, K.T.J. and Meltzer, D., 2019. The ImPreSS trial: implementation of point-of-care pharmacogenomic decision support in perioperative care. *Clinical pharmacology and therapeutics*, 106(6), p.1179.

UK Biobank, 2023. https://www.ukbiobank.ac.uk/learn-more-about-uk-biobank (accessed 21 May 2024).

van der Wouden, C.H., Böhringer, S., Cecchin, E., Cheung, K.C., Dávila-Fajardo, C.L., Deneer, V.H., Dolžan, V., Ingelman-Sundberg, M., Jönsson, S., Karlsson, M.O. and Kriek, M.,

2020. Generating evidence for precision medicine: considerations made by the Ubiquitous Pharmacogenomics Consortium when designing and operationalizing the PREPARE study. *Pharmacogenetics and Genomics*, *30*(6), pp.131–144.

Weiler, N., 2018. https://www.ucsf.edu/news/2018/03/410041/genomic-analysis-reveals-why-asthma-inhalers-fail-minority-children (accessed 13 August 2024).

Willis, 2024. https://pharmaceutical-journal.com/article/news/one-quarter-of-patients-in-pharmacogenomics-trial-have-had-prescriptions-changed (accessed 16 December 2024).

Youssef, E., Buck, J. and Wright, D., 2020. Understanding pharmacogenomic testing and its role in medicine prescribing. *Nursing Standard*, *35*(7), pp.55–60.

CHAPTER 8

Genomics, pharmacogenomics and the future

Chapter outline

This chapter considers the future of genomics and pharmacogenomics in terms of the impact of scientific developments on UK health care and the evolution of the nursing role to support the integration of genomics into health services.

Introduction

As our understanding of the biological basis of disease expands, genomics is advancing rapidly towards the point at which it is no longer seen as a specialist area and is becoming part of all health care. These are exciting times in which the technology is available to reveal genomic information about individuals which can improve health outcomes and increase patient safety for all. However, to realise the benefits of genomic medicine for patients, the NHS must keep pace with the momentum of scientific discovery and available genomics technologies must become fully integrated into services. The UK NHS is a world leader in genomic medicine but progress remains to be made in terms of the effective embedding of genomics into care pathways. Plans are in place to precipitate positive change, for example a strategic focus on increased and streamlined collaboration between pathology services and oncology services to support more extensive genomic testing in cancer care (NHS England, 2022).

Nurses will be essential to the effective integration of genomics and pharmacogenomics into health services (Calzone et al., 2018). Services embarking on this process require a prepared workforce and the nursing community must develop genomics skills and knowledge to help them deliver effective genomics care. Nurses must acquire the skills to identify genomic risk, discuss risk with patients and refer people to the right services, leading to quicker and more accurate diagnosis and safer and more effective treatment options. Many settings, including primary care settings, already facilitate the identification of genetic risk within their services, for example in relation to the provision of HRT and contraception. When taking a family health history as part of a consultation, practice nurses will ask questions which can lead to the identification of a pathogenic BRCA gene mutation within a woman's family and may precipitate referral to specialist genomics service. Nurses recording these details must be able to discuss suspected risk factors, any further actions and their implications competently to gain the confidence of patients. Nurses can also access the National Genomic Test Directory to check patient eligibility for specific tests to further inform discussion.

Care pathways are changing to incorporate obtaining and recording genetic and genomic information and the outcomes of any referrals within routine care pathways. Streamlining services in this way will facilitate the prompt identification of inherited pathogenic variants leading to adult-onset conditions including some complex conditions such as diabetes and cardiovascular disease, some types of cancer and cancer pre-disposition syndromes such as Lynch syndrome.

Nurses are the largest group of health care practitioners. They interact frequently with patients and are in a pivotal position to lead changes in ethical practice (Whitley et al., 2020). All nurses will need general knowledge of genomic medicine in the UK, but nurses in specialist areas will require specialist skills in this area. In addition to the testing process, nurses in areas where genomics is integrated into care need to have an awareness of common challenges associated with genomics, for example ethical issues linked to privacy and confidentiality when sharing genetic information within families. Nurses equipped with the skills required to discuss and manage ethical concerns can provide effective support and improve the patient experience.

Medicines are the biggest intervention in health care and as pharmacogenomic testing becomes integrated into practice, nurses administering medications as part of their role must keep abreast of changes in practice and adopt or design new pathways to improve medicines safety where possible (Hetland et al., 2024). Pharmacogenomics can help to mitigate the risk of adverse drug reactions. Refining what is known and its utility in relation to established drug–gene pairs alongside the development and integration of pre-treatment screening tests for many more drugs will improve nurses' abilities to optimise medicines regimes for patients.

The ability to request pre-treatment screening tests to obtain results quickly and to access information at any time from any previous pharmacogenomic tests will enable prescribers to maximise the advantages offered by genomics including a reduction in inappropriate prescribing or polypharmacy (Royal College of Physicians and British Pharmacological Society, 2022). Point of care pharmacogenomic testing is in its infancy but developing and implementing this type of testing where it is needed will help nurses to achieve immediate improvements in the safety and efficacy of many treatments. The next significant steps in the future integration of pharmacogenomics are for whole genome sequencing and pre-emptive medicines safety testing panels to become part of routine practice (Peruzzi et al., 2023).

The UK government's national genomics strategy spans three pillars:

■ *Diagnosis and personalised medicine* – to support the incorporation of genomic advances into services to improve diagnosis, stratification and treatment of disease. This concerns the embedding of genomics to improve care in areas such as cancer care, rare and inherited disease and infectious disease. It also considers how pharmacogenomic-guided treatment can be increased.

- *Prevention* – to enable predictive and preventive care to improve public health. This includes further development of early life, reproductive and adult screening.
- *Research* – to support vital research and the translation of findings into health care. This pillar outlines considerations for effective patient recruitment, data management and equality and diversity in research (UK Government, 2020).

Continued and sustained focus in these three areas will support the UK's trajectory towards individualised care for every patient. Current research pilots integrating genomics into routine health care, for example setting up new pharmacogenomics testing services, will enable the identification of foreseeable challenges and consideration of how these might be addressed. Aspects of the three core pillars are at various stages of development nationally. There have been strategic lessons to learn from the experiences of other countries integrating genomics into their health services, for example the Netherlands, which led the way on integrating DPD testing prior to fluoropyrimidine use to avoid toxicity in patients with genetic polymorphisms (Peruzzi et al., 2023). The UK followed in 2020, and this implementation in turn provided learning to inform wider national pharmacogenomic test rollout (Royal College of Physicians and British Pharmacological Society, 2022).

Media reports about scientific advances raise both public awareness and expectations regarding genomics in health care (Kirk et al., 2011). Many people now understand what whole genome sequencing (WGS) means and are aware of the potential to predict future health and improve health outcomes. The global implications of scientific development, however, include inequity of access between regions or between ethnic groups in all countries. In wealthier countries, there are risks associated with access to private genomic testing and the lack of support for individuals accessing direct to consumer tests and receiving problematic results.

Research and scientific momentum

Research continues into the genetic contribution to many diseases with the regular introduction of many breakthrough studies. In 2024, Oxford Nanopore started work on the world's first 'epigenetic map'. The study will analyse 50,000 DNA samples from UK Biobank to record modifications to gene expression. It is hope that the resulting dataset will provide new insights into diseases such as cancer and dementia (UK Government, 2025).

Genomic medicine is continuously discovering new connections between disease, the genome and precision treatments (NHS England, 2022). The field has evolved significantly over the past 20 years and genomic research has received significant increased focus and investment. For example, a government press release in 2022, announced a £175 million allocation to fund the 'most advanced genomic health care system in the world' (UK Government, 2022).

The use of computational methods such as artificial intelligence (AI) in genomics can help researchers to improve their understanding of patterns within genomic data sets. A genomic AI network of excellence, commissioned by NHS England, helps scientists to understand the opportunities and challenges involved. The network is collaborating with KiTEC, a health technology assessment team at King's College London with expertise in the evaluation of AI technologies in health care, to survey those working in genomics to capture their perspectives. This will inform progress and help pinpoint what is required to introduce AI safely and effectively into genomic medicine (NHS England, 2024).

In addition to scientific discovery and the creation of new technologies, the NHS must continue to review the efficacy of current technologies and identify where further research is needed. For example, in 2023, NICE conducted a health technology evaluation of the testing kit for MT-RNR1 variants in babies admitted to SCBU who will receive gentamicin. The evaluation explored factors such as:

- how the test affects time to antibiotics outside of neonatal intensive care units;
- how test results affect antibiotic prescribing;
- the failure rate of the test; and
- the diagnostic accuracy of the test.

Evaluation of the effectiveness of tests and associated changes in care enables regulation of developments to help ensure continued benefits and patient safety.

Targeted treatment

It is common for the national media to report on the successful use of new treatments. Headlines in 2023 included the story of Teddi, the first baby to receive gene therapy for metachromatic leukodystrophy. The treatment involved the removal of a faulty gene from the child's stem cells enabling her to lead a normal life (NHS England, 2023 B).

Other targeted treatments include gene editing technology such as CRIPSR (clustered regularly interspaced short palindromic repeats), which has the potential to correct genetic mutations prior to implanting an *in vitro* fertilised embryo (Connors and Schorn, 2018). The ability to use such treatments necessitates change within existing care pathways and previously separate services to become linked. Nurses practising in such services will require additional skills and knowledge alongside adaptability to change.

👓 New hope

Doctors at Moorfields eye hospital have recently been able to provide 'life changing' improvements to four children with severe childhood blindness trialling an experimental gene therapy.

The treatment involved injecting healthy copies of a faulty gene into the back of the eye.

Some of the children, whose vision had deteriorated since birth as a result of the genetic variant, could only distinguish between light and dark, but following the treatment, their parents reported that they had started to be able to draw and write (Mundasad, 2025).

Developments in gene-editing technologies continue to lead to new treatments for genetic conditions. A number of ongoing trials include those for CRISPR-based therapies such as Casgevy (exagamglogene autotemcel) for sickle cell disease, licensed in 2023. Research also continues into the development of a CRISPR technique that has an effect on methylation (chemical or 'methyl' grouping on a gene which influences gene expression). Genes can be edited to add or remove methyl groups. A clinical trial, started in 2024, is conducting research on the editing of the epigenome to add methylation and reverse gene expression to prevent muscular dystrophy (Brazil, 2024). This condition is sometimes caused by the absence of methylation on a gene usually only expressed in embryos, causing its continued expression.

The sequencing of tumour DNA has enabled the use of precision anti-cancer treatment, such as PARP inhibitors and immunotherapy or chemotherapy, but the search for new genotype-directed therapies continues. A large volume of current resource is dedicated to research on targeted therapies for non-small-cell lung cancer. Recent trials, including the National Lung Matrix Trial, involve the screening of tumours for several variants and allocating patients to appropriate treatments. Programmes such as this can be supported by embedding them into NHS practice, also requiring additional facets to the nursing role (Middleton et al., 2020).

The University of Oxford is leading on the Lynchvax project, funded by Cancer Research UK. This research aims to develop a vaccine for people with Lynch syndrome, which is the most common global cause of genetic cancers (Cancer Research UK, 2024).

Pharmacogenomics in the future

In addition to the genomics AI network, 'pharmacogenomics and medicines optimisation' represents another of the eight new NHS Genomic Networks of Excellence, bringing patients and clinical, academic and industry experts together to support genomics developments in UK health services. The networks are to be created as part of the first NHS genomics strategy and pharmacogenomics and medicines optimisation aims to address ineffective prescribing and to reduce adverse drug reactions (NHS England, 2024).

Some tests performed in secondary care, for example the CYP2C19 test to identify polymorphisms prior to clopidogrel use following acute stroke, may provide information at the point of care to inform clinical decision-making. Information from such tests will also have relevance for an individual's ongoing primary care throughout their lifetime and the future prescribing of other medicines with known or suspected drug–gene pairs, such as statins, proton pump inhibitors (PPIs) and selective serotonin reuptake inhibitors (SSRIs). In order to support the mainstreaming of pharmacogenomic services, health records must adapt to be able to facilitate the sharing of information relevant to prescribing decisions throughout health care teams. This necessitates the improved co-ordination of services and development of the means to overcome existing challenges associated with sharing health information between systems (Shepherd, 2016).

📖 **Learning activity**

- Design a hypothetical study to conduct research into drug–gene pairs for PPIs. Think about the data you will need to collect and how you will record and analyse it. You will also need to consider and provide a rationale for the inclusion and exclusion criteria for recruiting study participants.
- Consider any risks associated with your study and how you will protect study participants from harm.
- Design an information sheet to be given to people who are prescribed statins by their GP. The sheet will need to contain enough information to enable people to decide whether or not they wish to participate in the study. This might include aspects such as how samples will be obtained and how participants' personal information will be kept private.

Pre-emptive pharmacogenomic panel testing has great potential to improve care, but targeted research must be conducted to address unanswered questions regarding cost-effectiveness. Further data are also required to improve pharmacogenomic knowledge related to regimes of multiple medications, drug–gene pairs in non-European populations and rare genetic polymorphisms (Peruzzi et al., 2023). Global research has highlighted the necessity for increased data from diverse populations to enable ethical implementation of pharmacogenomics to benefit care nationally and internationally (Magavern et al., 2021). Lack of diversity has prompted recommendations that national pharmacogenomic services should receive funding to explore and address associated ethical, legal and social issues and ensure from the outset that provision does not exacerbate existing health inequalities (Pirmohamed, 2023).

Genome wide association studies use large numbers of DNA profiles to gain knowledge about the genetic contribution to specific diseases. It is important to look at the DNA of large numbers of people to research the genetic causes of individual responses to medicines. Although such studies can be expensive owing to the resources required, more of them are needed to identify variants caused by loss of function alleles that predispose individuals to adverse drug reactions (Cheek, 2017).

Multiple consortia have been established to research specific drug–gene pairs, including 'Metformin Genetics' and both the 'Individual Warfarin' and the 'Individual Clopidogrel' pharmacogenetics consortia. However, an increase in the number and the diversity of studies is required to continue to build the knowledge base and to translate findings effectively into clinical prescribing support (Peruzzi et al., 2023). The right information can help prescribers, including nurse prescribers, to select the most appropriate drug as the first line treatment and to make dosing decisions easier. More accessible decision support tools, for example related to precision dosing, would also better support the translation of research into prescribing practice (Magavern et al., 2021).

⚙️ Thinking point

Implementing pharmacogenomics across the NHS – key needs.
   Which of the following do you think the nursing community could contribute to?

- funding services;
- designing services;
- providing supporting laboratory infrastructure;
- providing clinical governance;
- standardising the consent process for pharmacogenomic tests;
- enabling health care record systems to support the sharing of results;
- improving the pharmacogenomics competence and confidence of prescribers; and
- maintaining and building patient and public trust in the NHS Genomic Medicine Service (Royal College of Physicians and British Pharmacological Society, 2022).

Pharmacogenomics is also vital for effective anti-microbial stewardship. Monitoring the effects of antimicrobials, by tracking levels of pathogens or a patient's biological response to an infection, can reveal whether antibiotics are effective and reduce unnecessary use (Blackburn et al., 2020).

> ### 🦉 Knowledge focus – anti-microbial stewardship
>
> To achieve effective antibiotics for future use, all nurses can:
>
> - follow standard principles of infection prevention and control;
> - be aware of local and national anti-microbial stewardship campaigns;
> - signpost patients to appropriate services and resources to minimise infections, for example sexual health services and travel vaccination clinics;
> - appropriately monitor patients on antibiotics for side effects;
> - review patients on antibiotics and assess the need for continued treatment; and
> - educate patients about anti-microbial resistance.
>
>   And nurse prescribers can:
>
> - follow local antibiotic treatment formularies;
> - obtain microbiological samples prior to prescribing antibiotics;
> - prescribe the narrowest spectrum antibiotic indicated for the shortest recommended amount of time;
> - review response to intravenous antibiotics within 48 hours and switch to oral antibiotics where possible; and
> - avoid repeat antimicrobial prescriptions (BNF, 2024).

The continued development and integration of genomics and pharmacogenomics into UK health services

NHS England stated in 2022, that over the following three years the NHS genomic laboratory hubs, genomic medicine service alliances and clinical genomics services would continue to transform clinical pathways and service models to embed genomics in settings where there is the greatest impact on clinical outcomes and pathway efficiencies (NHS England, 2022). This has included the following:

New infrastructure

New specialist pathology centres are being set up at major hub hospitals in each region. The evolution of the NovaSeq sequencing system allows the processing of greater volumes of data and creates more testing potential within the NHS (Modi et al., 2021). However, increased resources are required to support increased testing, interpretation of results and ongoing care. Genomic pathways in hospitals must be supported by a genomic-competent workforce. Effective connections must also be in place between specialist centres and labs so that samples, for example pathology samples from operating theatres, can be transported quickly and safely. Appropriate infrastructure and streamlined processes support collaboration between different settings to deliver timely and accurate test results (Middleton et al., 2020).

Increased services and improved access to services

The NHS also strives to achieve equity of access to services (NHS England, 2022) and a focus on unmet need by the NHS Genomic Medicine Service has precipitated an increase in services and support for rare diseases. Queen Elizabeth Hospital in Birmingham was the first UK hospital to offer virtual exercise classes for patients with

Pompe disease. This condition is a rare genetic metabolic disorder where problems with glycogen storage can lead to progressive muscle weakness, causing pain and fatigue. Physiotherapy can help to manage symptoms of Pompe disease, but it can prove difficult for patients from the wide geographical areas served by the hospital to attend. Online classes provide the opportunity for physiotherapy and for patients to connect with others with the condition (NHS, University Hospitals Birmingham, 2024).

This drive for better services and better access to services is reflected in other examples, such as cardiac care. A specialist nurse for inherited cardiac conditions (ICC) in the North of England has led research to help services for cardiomyopathy to meet patient need and to provide an improved patient experience. Empirical data showed that patients were not receiving adequate or timely information and support related to testing, diagnosis, treatment or discharge from services, leading to the implementation of key recommendations for improved patient communication (Goodfellow et al., 2020).

The management of inherited cardiac conditions requires a multidisciplinary approach to improve access to services and meet growing demand. Demand has risen owing to geographic variation in the areas covered by services and a lack of standardised care pathways. Inherited cardiac condition centres regularly need to link with other cardiology settings within a patient's care such as imaging, surgery and pathology and health care practitioners must practice collaboratively. Providing patients with equal access to services is a challenge in the current economic climate and nurse-led clinics have the potential to improve resource efficiency and to meet increased need. This model will benefit patients and their families for whom any diagnosis of ICC has implications and has been shown to be effective within familial hypercholesterolaemia (a sub-group of ICCs) services (Alway et al., 2024).

Nurses work across health systems and can reduce disparities in care by identifying where they occur and contributing to policy change. The majority of equity issues are related to inequitable access to genomics services among diverse ethnic groups, particularly in poorer or rural communities, and nurses in clinical services must take responsibility for adopting effective strategies to increase access in these areas. Such strategies include demonstrating effective leadership and advocacy for genomics services, using tools to trigger appropriate referrals, engaging in genomic risk prevention initiatives and creating accessible resources (Limoges et al., 2024). Improved access to testing services can also improve the diversity of genomic data in databases and their interpretive value and so it is important that nurse understand the social, cultural and financial contributors to disparities in order to try to address them (Sharif et al., 2020).

Modern health care

The relatively recent introduction of remote consultation has increased accessibility to relieve the current pressure on some services. This alternative mode of care delivery progressed in the Covid-19 era which necessitated a move to online health care. Remote pre-test counselling can improve access to services for some patients. Research shows a reduction in patient costs and time required for travel with a similar decrease in cost for health systems when patients are not required to attend a physical service (Danylchuk et al., 2021).

Private testing

Public awareness about the genetic determinants of health is growing (Carver et al., 2017). Better technology and increased availability also mean that genomic medicine is becoming more easily available for individuals to access independently. Elective genomic testing is a term used to describe individuals choosing to access a test to obtain genetic information without a medical indication and this can include whole genome sequencing. Such tests can be analysed to reveal personal health information independent of phenotype or family history but are not diagnostic. The information obtained could be used to inform future targeted screening or diagnostic tests.

Consumers should be aware that interpretation and reporting practices in terms of what is classified as a pathogenic or a likely pathogenic variant can vary between laboratories (Blout Zawatsky et al., 2022). Genetic counsellors and some nurses in specialist roles are trained to interpret and share results accurately and comprehensibly and the inability to interpret or the misinterpretation of private test results by individuals can lead to distress (Whitley et al., 2020). Patients receiving positive results for certain variants may experience severe anxiety but never go on to develop signs or symptoms. Some conditions have reduced penetrance, which means that not everybody within a population with a specific disease-causing genetic variation will go on to develop the disease. A common example is familial cancer syndromes where people with an inherited variant in the BRCA 1or BRCA 2 gene are at risk of developing cancer, but not all of them do.

Some direct-to-consumer (DTC) test companies offer polygenic risk scoring as part of their private testing process, even though this type of analysis has only recently begun to be standardised in clinical practice and scores cannot be quality assured (James et al., 2021). Notwithstanding limitations such as this, an awareness of the availability, prevalence, levels of accuracy and potential benefits of DTC genetic testing is important. Individuals who access private tests may proceed to share positive, uncertain or unclear results for interpretation and further action and nurses must be prepared to respond to questions about results from private tests and also to integrate these results into a patient's health records and ongoing care (Flowers et al., 2020).

Veritas (a genetic testing company) offers genetic testing for patients in China, but does not provide post-test counselling for patients. People accessing private tests may miss out on support to understand any associated challenges or to manage the potential impact of genomic test results on their lives and those of their families, and on valuable health advice from health care practitioners (Chair et al., 2019). Patient education has long been a part of the nursing role and nurses are well positioned to provide guidance about DTC testing. Nurses can also provide valuable contributions to address gaps in the evidence base related to patient experiences of private testing, which can be used to improve the experiences of others (Flowers et al., 2020).

📖 Learning activity

Look at the following company websites for information about which direct to consumer genetic and genomic tests are available online:

- Color (https://www.color.com/);
- 23 and me (https://www.23andme.com/);
- Cegat (https://cegat.com/).

Preparing the workforce

Not all health care professionals will need to develop expertise in genomics, but all professions must develop the genomic skills and knowledge relevant to their practice. In all nursing practice, basic biosciences is relevant knowledge and the identification of genetic or genomic risk and referring people to specialist genetic services when required is a relevant skill (NHS England, 2022). Additional essential skills include the ability to discuss genomics and genomics-related care competently with other practitioners in order to co-ordinate care between settings.

The Genomics Education Programme has developed a strategic framework to support the incorporation of genomics into pharmacist education and training (Health Education England, 2024A). This framework sets out a 3 year approach that will empower the pharmacy workforce to use genomic tools to support medicines optimisation and improve patient outcomes. The framework supports a multi-disciplinary approach to genomics-based care and recognises that shared skills and knowledge enable health care teams, including nurses, to meet patient needs. Genomics literacy must improve across all health care professions so that practitioners can work effectively together (Calzone et al., 2018).

Preparing the UK health workforce to deliver the digital future is vital, particularly in genomics where effective use of new technologies can transform care by reducing delayed diagnosis and preventing the 'diagnostic odyssey' experienced by many patients or parents of patients with genetic conditions (Health Education England, 2019; Health Education England, 2024C). The NHS Genomic Medicine Service is integral to professional development. This service provides training resources and online learning, and funding for masters' programmes for NHS staff, and raises awareness for example through initiatives such as the annual 'Genomics Conversation Week' (NHS England, 2022).

Genomic medicine and the role of the nurse

In all nursing roles, nurses must assess patients and then plan and implement high-quality person-centred care (RCN, 2024). Taking a family health history is part of a comprehensive assessment and as NHS genomic infrastructure expands and new systems are established, genomic testing will become part of a larger number of routine care pathways. Nurses must be ready to adopt innovations in practice such as point of care tests and to acquire the skills to ensure that the care they provide meets patient needs and realises the benefits offered by genomic testing (Buaki-Sogo and Percival, 2022).

Registered nurses working in key genomics areas will require specialist training towards developing their practice and the genomics training academy for specialist nurses, part of the Genomics Education Programme, provides online and in-person education for the UK genomics laboratory and clinical workforce (Health Education England, 2024B).

The oncology setting represents a good example of an area where genomics is utilised routinely for testing and treatment. System changes are well established, the testing of tumour DNA supports precision oncology and pharmacogenomic information enables the safer use of chemotherapy drugs and a better patient experience. There is very little evidence on how genomics and pharmacogenomics are impacting on the nursing role, but the biggest contributions so far have been provided by cohorts of oncology nurses (Hetland et al., 2024). Nurses must be equipped to 'socialise' patients with genomics and its associated issues and information and transparency will empower people to make decisions around risk, ethics, privacy, insurance, employment and fertility (Health Education England, 2018, p.20).

Nurse leadership

Nurses support patients in every aspect of their care and so the nursing contribution to health policy is vital for improving services for patients (Calzone et al., 2010). Nurses can help to raise awareness of the benefits of genomics and provide direction in the establishing of effective care for patients on their genomics journeys. Leadership skills for nurses will be important in bringing about and driving organisational change towards high standards of care. Nurse leaders should consider effective strategies for engaging the nursing workforce and for promoting clinical competence in genomics at all levels (Kirk et al., 2011).

As genomics is integrated into different clinical areas there will be many challenges, including different organisational levels of commitment, organisational culture, internal and external politics and financial status. These are barriers that nurse leaders must address in order to transform services. The Global Genomics Nursing Alliance has provided a Roadmap for Global Acceleration of Genomics Integration across nursing which can be adapted across diverse settings to provide a practical and coordinated approach. The roadmap helps nurse leaders to ask the right questions to inform planning. Stages of integration include identifying stakeholders, allocating resources and evaluating progress to help ensure the success of any changes (Tonkin et al., 2020).

To attain optimal outcomes within individual clinical settings, nurses must be involved in decisions about how care will be delivered, and associated practical, legal and ethical considerations such as how patient privacy and confidentiality will be protected. Nurses must be allowed to share their insights to produce clear and effective practice guidelines. As part of any organisational change, the nursing workforce should identify and ask for the education they need to achieve additional proficiencies. They must be assertive in negotiating what is required for them to practice effectively (Jenkins, 2011.)

📖 Learning activity

Six critical success factors have been outlined for the effective integration of genomics into health services. These are:

1. health care transformation;
2. education and training;
3. effective nursing practice;
4. sustainable infrastructure and resources;
5. collaboration and communication; and
6. patient and public involvement (Tonkin et al., 2020).

- ■ Imagine you are planning to address each of these factors and identify some key considerations. These might be related to resources, variables or data.
- ■ Write a list of recommendations to achieve successful integration of genomics in terms of 'effective nursing practice'.

Nursing and research

Nursing research on the benefits and outcomes of genomics care can inform the development of future provision (Calzone et al., 2010). Nurses have conducted research into specific areas, for example into some of the ethical issues related to genomics and findings from these studies have contributed to ethical guidance. For example, disparities in access to care or health outcomes can result from ethnicity or gender and nurses are well placed to make a significant difference through research into reducing health disparities (Conley and Tinkle, 2007).

It has long been recognised that nurses provide a unique perspective of health which, in addition to the biological viewpoint, is valuable to genomics research in terms of behavioural, social and ethical considerations. In the UK, our increasing capability to identify population sub-groups who may experience health inequality but will benefit from genomic medicine is improving risk prevention (Kirk et al., 2011). Nurses should be supported by appropriate education and inter-disciplinary collaboration to contribute to genomics research where possible and increasing participation in under-represented groups can help reduce health inequities (Limoges et al., 2024). The Improving Black Health Outcomes is a new research initiative from the NIHR BioResource and Kings College London, which studies health conditions disproportionately affecting Black communities. Participation will contribute to future strategies to meet need and improve outcomes for Black individuals (NIHR, 2024).

Nurses have important roles in trialling new treatments for genetic conditions, for example gene therapies. They must ensure patients have the information they require at every stage of treatment and that the effects of new treatments are monitored carefully. They must also navigate managing and sharing trial data in accordance with research ethics and the law. Following extensive trials, new medicines and new technologies are being approved and licensed for use in practice. Nurses can make a significant difference in the effective embedding of genomic medicine into clinical practice for the benefit of patients by supporting the integration of these new technologies effectively into care pathways (Conley and Tinkle 2007).

Nurse education

Nurse education providers must keep pace with developments in practice in order to equip newly qualified nurses with the skills and knowledge required to maximise the potential of genomics technology and infrastructure (Calzone et al., 2018). Chapter 3 explores the core skills and knowledge required for nursing genomic literacy. However, recent research shows that some health care professionals consider themselves to have low levels of genomic literacy. Nurses are required to understand key genomic and pharmacogenomic principles but significant barriers to the provision of meaningful genomic education include cost and a lack of vital resources such as nurse educators who feel competent and confident to teach genomics (Whitley et al., 2020; Connors and Schorn, 2018).

Nurses who understand DNA structure and function have an increased awareness of how genetic variation can affect health. Nurses at all levels must have the ability to take a family history, to identify patient and family genomic risk and to make necessary referrals. It is also necessary for nurses to learn about the national genomic testing infrastructure to provide accurate information about accessing tests, and to have an awareness of the benefits and limitations of genomics to inform initial discussion. Education about the ethical and legal issues related to sharing information is crucial to nursing practice, for example giving patient and family information effectively while protecting the privacy of others and protecting data in line with General Data Protection Regulation. It is also useful to prepare for experiences such as managing results from direct-to-consumer tests if presented (Daack-Hirsch et al., 2011).

Inconsistency in the quality and extent of pre-registration education between providers has occurred owing to a lack of agreed national standards, learning outcomes and guidelines for educators (Kirk et al., 2011). Competency frameworks have gone some way towards addressing this issue, including the UK 2023 nursing competency framework (NHS England, 2023A). The American 'Essentials of Genetic and Genomic Nursing: Competencies, Curricula guidelines and Outcome Indicators' (Consensus Panel, 2008) also includes outcome indicators to enable educators to determine when a specific competency has been achieved. Effective international collaboration can support the development of the global nursing community in genomics. A study by Chair et al. (2019) found that mainland China, Hong Kong and Taiwan could learn from the UK and the US regarding the development of genomics competencies for nurses.

In addition to the level and type of knowledge required, it is also imperative for educators to consider how they can secure practice placements which help students to apply skills, such as giving patient information effectively, and to develop readiness for practice (Connors and Schorn, 2018). This means that practice assessors (registrants who support student development in clinical areas) must be confident to support students in genomics learning and to answer their questions. Access to up-to-date information and to training is essential for the continued professional development of qualified staff (Kirk et al., 2011). Without this, the gap between the genomic proficiency of students graduating today and that of those who joined the register before completion of the human genome project will continue to widen (Donnelly et al., 2017). Since 2011, the online Genomics Education Programme has continued to grow and provides resources for nurses at all levels. Chapter 3 lists some other resources to support registered nurses to integrate genomics into their practice.

📖 Learning activity

■ List five examples of episodes of care which could provide the opportunity for a student nurse to extend their knowledge of genomics.

Global communities

Genomics has the potential to reduce global health inequalities by providing low-income countries with cost-effective methods of treating and preventing major diseases, but this will prove successful only when resources are distributed to all countries. There is a greater volume of reported disease and an increased number of health issues in developing nations but both funding for medical research and treatment options discovered through genomic research are predominantly available in richer countries (WHO, 2020). Genomics enables health care practitioners to meet population health needs through targeted screening, accurate diagnosis and timely therapeutic intervention (Calzone et al., 2010) however, disparate political and financial positions in countries across the world can curb inherent possibilities.

The stage of integration of genomics technology into health systems and care varies across the globe. In any country, a framework which involves the effective use of nursing knowledge, or 'intellectual capital' can support good nursing practice. The following key principles can be applied to genomics to influence both organisational and patient outcomes:

1. building and consolidating knowledge and skills of individual nurses through academic preparation and continued professional development;
2. development of and access to practice resources, guidelines and local protocols; and
3. establishing relationships and networks to share best practice between colleagues (Ridge et al., 2022).

Effective, clinically relevant genomics resources are important to support both nurses and nurse educators, and shared repositories can help to resolve variations in proficiency and to standardise care in different countries (Calzone et al., 2018). The international society of genomics nurses (ISONG, https://www.isong.org/) has a repository of resources in English for registered nurses.

Whole genome sequencing

Completed in 2018, the 100,000 genomes project made groundbreaking progress for exploring the utility of whole genome sequencing in practice. However, in the clinical setting, whole genome sequencing still requires the application of virtual panels for the analysis (Buaki-Sogo and Percival, 2022). Exploring what would be required to achieve the introduction of whole genome sequencing within the NHS to inform clinical care is included in the NHS England (2022) strategy to accelerate genomic medicine in the UK. The Generation Study, launched in 2023, began making further strides towards recognising how individual whole genome sequencing at birth might become a reality.

This study is assessing the utility and feasibility of screening newborns for a larger number of child onset conditions than the current newborn blood spot screening. Umbilical blood samples from 100,000 babies at a range of sites, which include diverse and underserved populations, are tested for more than 200 conditions that usually appear in early life. Tests cover conditions that can be treated within the UK if identified early. It was predicted that 1% of babies would have positive results from screening and go on to have further diagnostic tests, and Genetic Alliance UK can support clinicians to manage these cases (Genomics England, 2024).

Genomics England is working in partnership with the NHS to explore how genomic data can be used and the risks and benefits of storing genomic data over an individual's lifetime. Health data from The Generation Study and from Our Future Health (2024), a study exploring genomics and population health, will be added to the National Genomic Research library and pharmaceutical companies will be able to pay to access this data.

Collecting information to inform future care is vital and the US has created a genetic test registry (https://www.ncbi.nlm.nih.gov/gtr/) where practitioners can submit genetic test information, such as tests requested, how they were performed and how the results were used to inform care, to contribute to the growing picture of the genetic basis of health and disease.

⚕ My condition, my DNA

The Genetic Alliance UK Patient Charter: Recommendations for the integration of Whole Genome Sequencing into UK health services outlines the wishes of patients in relation to WGS:

1. Patients want the option to receive as much information about their health as possible from whole genome sequencing.
2. Patients value genetic counselling and are keen for the support of genetic counsellors before and after whole genome sequencing.
3. Patients welcome the sharing of their genomic data for research purposes.
4. Patients think that the NHS needs to make more progress towards preparing for the integration of whole genome sequencing into clinical practice (PET, 2015).

📖 Learning activity

■ Imagine you are going to take part in a debate. Prepare comprehensive 'for' and 'against' arguments for the introduction of national whole genome sequencing at birth in the UK.

(This learning activity is linked to NHS England (2023A) genomic nursing competency 6.)

Summary

In conjunction with rapid advances in technology, health systems are changing to integrate genomics into routine care and health care tailored to individuals' genetic profiles has become a reality (Connors and Schorn, 2018). To adapt to this new reality the role of health care practitioners is changing and nurses must develop new skills and knowledge, to ensure that they are genomics competent, research competent and culturally competent (Sharif et al., 2020). Transforming services is also creating opportunities for nurse leadership, but nurses will require support in the form of education and effective organisational and clinical governance to perform their roles safely, ethically and legally. In this way, nurses must be enabled to translate genomics education into practice and to continuously develop to support patients on their journeys and help them to face common challenges.

Despite the increasing availability of genomic technologies and the recognised clinical benefits of genomics and pharmacogenomics, there remain some significant obstacles associated with the integration of genomics into practice (Peruzzi et al., 2023). The NHS must develop the ability to make health information more available to underpin effective shared care and effective communication between services to meet patient needs.

As we continue to conduct research and to gather and analyse data, we will be better able to predict individual responses to medicines and to improve the safety of treatment and improve patient experience. The UK is a global leader in genomics, supported by effective national strategy as we continue on our path towards achieving personalised medicine and better health outcomes for all.

References

Alway, T., Bastiaenen, R., Pantazis, A., Robert, L., Akilapa, R., Whitaker, J., Page, S.P. and Carr-White, G., 2024. The development of inherited cardiac conditions services: current position and future perspectives. *British Medical Bulletin*, *150*(1), pp.11–22.

Blackburn L, Babb de Villiers C, Janus J et al. (2020) Genomic innovation: technologies for personalised medicine. www.ahsnnetwork.com/wp-content/uploads/2020/07/FINAL-AHSN-fullreport.pdf (accessed 29 August 2024).

Blout Zawatsky, C.L., Bick, D., Bier, L., Funke, B., Lebo, M., Lewis, K.L., Orlova, E., Qian, E., Ryan, L., Schwartz, M.L. and Soper, E.R., 2023. Elective genomic testing: practice resource of the National Society of Genetic Counselors. *Journal of Genetic Counseling*, *32*(2), pp.281–299.

BNF, 2024. Antimicrobial stewardship. https://bnf.nice.org.uk/medicines-guidance/antimicrobial-stewardship/#guidance-for-health-and-social-care-staff (accessed 9 September 2024).

Brazil, R., 2024. Targeting better safety: next steps for CRISPR therapeutics. https://pharmaceutical-journal.com/article/feature/targeting-better-safety-next-steps-for-crispr-therapeutics (accessed 4 October 2024).

Buaki-Sogo, M. and Percival, N., 2022. Genomic medicine: the role of the nursing workforce. *Nursing Times*, *118*, pp.1–3.

Calzone, K.A., Cashion, A., Feetham, S., Jenkins, J., Prows, C.A., Williams, J.K. and Wung, S.F., 2010. Nurses transforming health care using genetics and genomics. *Nursing Outlook*, *58*(1), pp.26–35.

Calzone, K.A., Kirk, M., Tonkin, E., Badzek, L., Benjamin, C. and Middleton, A., 2018. Increasing nursing capacity in genomics: overview of existing global genomics resources. *Nurse Education Today*, *69*, pp.53–59.

Cancer Research UK, 2024. News. https://news.cancerresearchuk.org/2024/09/10/lynchvax-cancer-vaccine-for-people-with-lynch-syndrome-funding/ (accessed 31 October 2024).

Carver, R.B., Castéra, J., Gericke, N., Evangelista, N.A.M. and El-Hani, C.N., 2017. Young adults' belief in genetic determinism, and knowledge and attitudes towards modern genetics and genomics: the PUGGS questionnaire. *PloS One*, *12*(1), p.e0169808.

Chair, S.Y., Waye, M.M.Y., Calzone, K. and Chan, C.W.H., 2019. Genomics education in nursing in Hong Kong, Taiwan and mainland China. *International Nursing Review*, *66*(4), pp.459–466.

Cheek, D.J., 2017. Pharmacogenomics: strategies for individualized *care. Nursing2020 Critical Care*, *12*(1), pp.22–27.

Conley, Y.P. and Tinkle, M.B., 2007. The future of genomic nursing research. *Journal of Nursing Scholarship*, *39*(1), pp.17–24.

Connors, L. and Schorn, M., 2018. Genetics and genomics content in nursing education: a national imperative. *Journal of Professional Nursing: Official Journal of the American Association of Colleges of Nursing*, *34*(4), pp.235–237.

Daack-Hirsch, S., Dieter, C. and Quinn Griffin, M.T., 2011. Integrating genomics into undergraduate nursing education. *Journal of Nursing Scholarship*, *43*(3), pp.223–230.

Danylchuk, N.R., Cook, L., Shane-Carson, K.P., Cacioppo, C.N., Hardy, M.W., Nusbaum, R., Steelman, S.C. and Malinowski, J., 2021. Telehealth for genetic counseling: a systematic evidence review. *Journal of Genetic Counseling*, *30*(5), pp.1361–1378.

Donnelly, M.K., Nersesian, P.V., Foronda, C., Jones, E.L. and Belcher, A.E., 2017. Nurse faculty knowledge of and confidence in teaching genetics/genomics: implications for faculty development. *Nurse Educator*, *42*(2), pp.100–104.

Flowers, E., Leutwyler, H. and Shim, J.K., 2020. Direct-to-consumer genomic testing: are nurses prepared? *Nursing2023*, *50*(8), pp.48–52.

Genomics England, 2024. Newborn Genomes programme. https://www.genomicsengland. co.uk/initiatives/newborns (accessed 5 September 2024).

Goodfellow, J., Stark, C., Mackersie, I. and Mackersie, V., 2020. 'Sometimes you just need someone to guide you through the maze' – improving cardiac care services in the North of England: suggestions from a patient-led project. *British Journal of Cardiac Nursing*, 15(2), pp.1–12.

Health Education England, 2019 The Topol review: Preparing the workforce to deliver the digital future. https://topol.hee.nhs.uk/wp-content/uploads/HEE-Topol-Review-2019.pdf

Health Education England, 2024A. News. https://www.genomicseducation.hee.nhs.uk/news/new-framework-for-upskilling-the-pharmacy-workforce-in-genomics/ (accessed 21 August 2024).

Health Education England, 2024B. GTAC: the genomics training academy. https://www. genomicseducation.hee.nhs.uk/about-us/gtac/ (accessed 31 August 2024).

Health Education England 2024-C. Diagnostic odyssey in rare disease. https://www. genomicseducation.hee.nhs.uk/genotes/knowledge-hub/the-diagnostic-odyssey-in-rare-disease/

Hetland, L.H., Maguire, J., Debono, D. and Wright, H., 2024. Scholarly literature on nurses and pharmacogenomics: a scoping review. *Nurse Education Today*, 137, p.106153.

James, J.E., Riddle, L., Koenig, B.A. and Joseph, G., 2021. The limits of personalization in precision medicine: polygenic risk scores and racial categorization in a precision breast cancer screening trial. *PLoS One*, 16(10), p.e0258571.

Jenkins, J., 2011, February. Essential genetic and genomic nursing competencies for the oncology nurse. *Seminars in Oncology Nursing*, 27(1), pp.64–71.

Kirk, M., Campalani, S., Doris, F., Heron, J., Mannion, G., Metcalfe, A., Patch, C., Permalloo, N., Shepherd, M. and Calzone, K., 2011. Genetics/genomics in nursing and midwifery: Task and Finish Group report to the nursing and midwifery professional advisory board. https:// assets.publishing.service.gov.uk/media/5a7cb326ed915d63cc65c50d/dh_131947.pdf

Limoges, J., Chiu, P., Dordunoo, D., Puddester, R., Pike, A., Wonsiak, T., Zakher, B., Carlsson, L. and Mussell, J.K., 2024. Nursing strategies to address health disparities in genomic informed care: a scoping review. *JBI Evidence Synthesis*,

Magavern, E.F., Daly, A.K., Gilchrist, A. and Hughes, D., 2021. Pharmacogenomics spotlight commentary: from the United Kingdom to global populations. *British Journal of Clinical Pharmacology*, 87(12), 4546–4548.

Middleton, G., Fletcher, P., Popat, S., Savage, J., Summers, Y., Greystoke, A., Gilligan, D., Cave, J., O'rourke, N., Brewster, A. and Toy, E., 2020. The National Lung Matrix Trial of personalized therapy in lung cancer. *Nature*, 583(7818), pp.807–812.

Modi, A., Vai, S., Caramelli, D. and Lari, M., 2021. The Illumina sequencing protocol and the NovaSeq 6000 system. In *Bacterial Pangenomics: Methods and Protocols*. New York: Springer, pp. 15–42.

Mundasad, 2025. 'Life-changing' gene therapy for children born blind. https://www.bbc.co.uk/ news/articles/c5ydnz2d75xo (accessed 11 March 2025).

NHS England, 2022. Accelerating genomic medicine in the NHS. https://www.england.nhs.uk/ long-read/accelerating-genomic-medicine-in-the-nhs/ (accessed 28 August 2024).

NHS England, 2023A. The 2023 genomic competency framework for UK nurses. https://www. genomicseducation.hee.nhs.uk/wp-content/uploads/2023/12/2023-Genomic-Competency-Framework-for-UK-Nurses.pdf

NHS England, 2023B. News. https://www.england.nhs.uk/2023/02/first-baby-receives-life-saving-gene-therapy-on-nhs/ (accessed 3 September 2024).

NHS England, 2024. Genomic networks of excellence. https://www.england.nhs.uk/genomics/ nhs-genomic-networks-of-excellence/#ai (accessed 4 September 2024).

NHS University Hospitals Birmingham, 2024. News. https://www.uhb.nhs.uk/news-and-events/news/patients-with-rare-disease-offered-uks-first-online-exercise-classes/634791 (accessed 29 August 2024).

NICE, 2023. Genedrive MT-RNR1 ID Kit for detecting a genetic variant to guide antibiotic use and prevent hearing loss in babies: early value assessment. https://www.nice.org.uk/guidance/hte6/chapter/Update-information (accessed 28 August 2024).

NIHR, 2024. Improving Black health outcomes https://bioresource.nihr.ac.uk/centres-programmes/improving-black-health-outcomes-ibho/ (accessed 31 October 2024).

Our Future Health, 2024. https://ourfuturehealth.org.uk/ (accessed 4 September 2024).

Consensus Panel and established by Outcome Indicators Consensus, 2008. *Essentials of genetic and genomic nursing: competencies, curricula guidelines, and outcome indicators.* American Nurses Association. https://www.genome.gov/Pages/Careers/HealthProfessionalEducation/geneticscompetency.pdf

Peruzzi, E., Roncato, R., De Mattia, E., Bignucolo, A., Swen, J.J., Guchelaar, H.J., Toffoli, G. and Cecchin, E., 2023. Implementation of pre-emptive testing of a pharmacogenomic panel in clinical practice: Where do we stand? *British Journal of Clinical Pharmacology*, *91*(2), pp.270–282.

PET, 2015. Genome sequencing: what do patients think? https://www.progress.org.uk/genome-sequencing-what-do-patients-think/ (accessed 3 October 2024).

Pirmohamed, M. (2023). Pharmacogenomics: current status and future perspectives. *Nature Reviews Genetics*, 24, 350–362.

RCN, 2024. Definition and principles of nursing. https://www.rcn.org.uk/Professional-Development/Definition-and-principles-of-nursing (accessed 6 March 2025).

Ridge, L.J., Liebermann, E.J., Stimpfel, A.W., Klar, R.T., Dickson, V.V. and Squires, A.P., 2022. The intellectual capital supporting nurse practice in a post-emergency state: a case study. *Journal of Advanced Nursing*, *78*(9), pp.3000–3011.

Royal College of Physicians and British Pharmacological Society, 2022. Joint Working Party. Personalised Prescribing: Using pharmacogenomics to improve outcomes. https://www.bps.ac.uk/getmedia/b43a3dca-1bbf-4bff-9379-20bef9349a8c/Personalised-prescribing-full-report.pdf.aspx

Sharif, S.M., Blyth, M., Ahmed, M., Sheridan, E., Saltus, R., Yu, J., Tonkin, E. and Kirk, M., 2020. Enhancing inclusion of diverse populations in genomics: a competence framework. *Journal of genetic counseling*, *29*(2), pp.282–292.

Shepherd, S., 2016. Coordinated care: a patient perspective on the impact of a fragmented system of care on experiences and outcomes, drawing on practical examples. *Future Healthcare Journal*, *3*(2), pp.136–138.

Tonkin, E., Calzone, K.A., Badzek, L., Benjamin, C., Middleton, A., Patch, C. and Kirk, M., 2020. A roadmap for global acceleration of genomics integration across nursing. *Journal of Nursing Scholarship*, *52*(3), pp.329–338.

UK Government, 2020. Genome UK: the future of healthcare. https://www.gov.uk/government/publications/genome-uk-the-future-of-healthcare (accessed 28 August 2024).

UK Government, 2022, News. https://www.gov.uk/government/news/over-175-million-for-cutting-edge-genomics-research (accessed 29 August 2024).

UK Government, 2025. News. https://www.gov.uk/government/news/landmark-genetics-partnership-to-probe-causes-of-cancer-and-dementia (accessed 11 March 2025).

Whitley, K.V., Tueller, J.A. and Weber, K.S., 2020. Genomics education in the era of personal genomics: academic, professional, and public considerations. *International journal of molecular sciences*, *21*(3), p.768.

WHO, 2020. Genomics. https://www.who.int/health-topics/genomics#tab=tab_1

Index

Note: Numbers in **bold** indicate tables, those in *italics* indicate figures.